Applying Corpus Linguistics to Illness and Healthcare

Communication is central to the experience of illness and the provision of healthcare. This book showcases the insights that can be gained into health communication by means of corpus linguistics – the computer-aided linguistic analysis of large datasets of naturally occurring language use known as *corpora*. The book takes readers through various stages of corpus linguistic research on health communication, from formulating research questions to disseminating findings to interested stakeholders. It helps readers anticipate and manage the different kinds of challenges they may encounter, and shows the variety of applications of the methods discussed, from interactions in Accident and Emergency departments to online discussions of mental illness and press representations of obesity. Providing the reader with a wide range of clear case studies, this book makes the relevant methods and findings accessible, engaging, and inspiring. This title is also available Open Access on Cambridge Core.

ELENA SEMINO is Distinguished Professor in the Department of Linguistics and English Language at Lancaster University, and Director of the ESRC Centre for Corpus Approaches to Social Science. She is a fellow of the UK's Academy of Social Sciences and has held visiting professorships at universities in China and Italy.

PAUL BAKER is Professor of Linguistics at Lancaster University. He has published widely on the application of corpus linguistics to the study of language, identity, and health. He has written 26 books, including *Using Corpora for Discourse Analysis* (2006), *The Language of Patient Feedback* (2019), and *Obesity in the News* (2021). He is the commissioning editor of the journal *Corpora*.

GAVIN BROOKES is Reader and UKRI Future Leader Fellow in the Department of Linguistics and English Language at Lancaster University. He has published widely using corpus linguistic, critical, and multimodal approaches to discourse analysis, with a particular focus on health(care) contexts.

LUKE COLLINS is Senior Research Associate with the ESRC Centre for Corpus Approaches to Social Science. His work is concerned with applications of corpus approaches in health communication contexts, and his research also addresses methodological challenges related to investigating digital discourses.

TONY MCENERY is Distinguished Professor of Linguistics and English Language in the Department of Linguistics and English Language at Lancaster University and Advisory Professor at Shanghai International Studies University in China. He has published widely on corpus linguistics, including *Corpus Linguistics* (with Hardie, 2011) and *Fundamental Principles of Corpus Linguistics* (with Brezina, 2022).

Applying Corpus Linguistics to Illness and Healthcare

Elena Semino
Lancaster University

Paul Baker
Lancaster University

Gavin Brookes
Lancaster University

Luke Collins
Lancaster University

Tony McEnery
Lancaster University

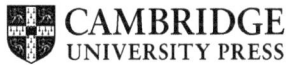

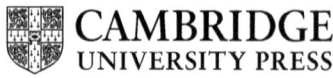
CAMBRIDGE
UNIVERSITY PRESS

Shaftesbury Road, Cambridge CB2 8EA, United Kingdom
One Liberty Plaza, 20th Floor, New York, NY 10006, USA
477 Williamstown Road, Port Melbourne, VIC 3207, Australia
314–321, 3rd Floor, Plot 3, Splendor Forum, Jasola District Centre,
New Delhi – 110025, India
103 Penang Road, #05–06/07, Visioncrest Commercial, Singapore 238467

Cambridge University Press is part of Cambridge University Press & Assessment, a department of the University of Cambridge.

We share the University's mission to contribute to society through the pursuit of education, learning and research at the highest international levels of excellence.

www.cambridge.org
Information on this title: www.cambridge.org/9781009477703

DOI: 10.1017/9781009477680

© Elena Semino, Paul Baker, Gavin Brookes, Luke Collins and Tony McEnery 2025

This publication is in copyright. Subject to statutory exception and to the provisions of relevant collective licensing agreements, with the exception of the Creative Commons version the link for which is provided below, no reproduction of any part may take place without the written permission of Cambridge University Press & Assessment.

An online version of this work is published at doi.org/10.1017/9781009477680 under a Creative Commons Open Access license CC-BY-NC 4.0 which permits re-use, distribution and reproduction in any medium for non-commercial purposes providing appropriate credit to the original work is given and any changes made are indicated. To view a copy of this license visit https://creativecommons.org/licenses/by-nc/4.0

When citing this work, please include a reference to the DOI 10.1017/9781009477680

First published 2025

A catalogue record for this publication is available from the British Library

A Cataloging-in-Publication data record for this book is available from the Library of Congress

ISBN 978-1-009-47770-3 Hardback
ISBN 978-1-009-47767-3 Paperback

Cambridge University Press & Assessment has no responsibility for the persistence or accuracy of URLs for external or third-party internet websites referred to in this publication and does not guarantee that any content on such websites is, or will remain, accurate or appropriate.

For EU product safety concerns, contact us at Calle de José Abascal, 56, 1°, 28003 Madrid, Spain, or email eugpsr@cambridge.org

Contents

List of Figures	*page* viii
List of Tables	ix
Acknowledgements	xi

1 Introduction 1
  1.1 Why This Book? 1
  1.2 An Overview of Corpus Linguistic Analytical Techniques 3
  1.3 The Structure of This Book 8

2 Research Questions 16
  2.1 Introduction 16
  2.2 Developing Exploratory Questions 17
  2.3 Developing Questions in Interaction with Stakeholders 20
  2.4 Working with a Set of Pregiven Questions from Non-academic Partners 25
  2.5 Conclusion 30

3 Collecting Data 33
  3.1 Introduction 33
  3.2 Compiling a News Corpus about Obesity 34
  3.3 Working with Pre-existing Transcript Data from Healthcare Settings 39
  3.4 Building a Historical Corpus of Anti-vaccination Literature 46
  3.5 Conclusion 52

4 Ethics 55
  4.1 Introduction 55
  4.2 Ethical Considerations When Studying Online Forums: Research on a Forum Dedicated to Pain 56
  4.3 Ethical Considerations When Working across Contexts and with Partners: Research on Public Discourses of Dementia 60
  4.4 Conclusion 65

5 Interaction 68
  5.1 Introduction 68
  5.2 Co-constructed Humour on a Forum for People with Cancer 69
  5.3 Sequences of Communicative Purposes in an Online Anxiety Support Forum 74
  5.4 Conclusion 82

6 Language Use and Identity 85
6.1 Introduction 85
6.2 Using Demographic Metadata 87
6.3 Using Mentions of Identity in the Data 93
6.4 Conclusion 97

7 Change over Time 101
7.1 Introduction 101
7.2 Patient Feedback: Identifying Increasing and Decreasing Lexical Items over Time 102
7.3 Representations of Obesity: Identifying Changing Topics over Time and Considering the Annual News Cycle 106
7.4 Anxiety Forum: Age and Level of Experience as Types of Time 112
7.5 Conclusion 116

8 Historical Data 118
8.1 Introduction 118
8.2 Anti-vaccination Discourse in Nineteenth-Century England 118
8.3 Representations around Sexually Transmitted Diseases in Early English Books Online 126
8.4 Conclusion 130

9 Representing the Experience of Illness 134
9.1 Introduction 134
9.2 Representing Anxiety 134
9.3 Representing Cancer 143
9.4 Conclusion 151

10 Representing Social Actors 153
10.1 Introduction 153
10.2 Representing Obesity in the British National Press 154
10.3 Investigating the Agency of Voices in Psychosis 160
10.4 Conclusion 167

11 Positions Legitimated 169
11.1 Introduction 169
11.2 Legitimation of Vaccine Hesitancy 170
11.3 Legitimation of Patient Evaluations of Healthcare Services 179
11.4 Conclusion 183

12 Dissemination 186
12.1 Introduction 186
12.2 Working with an External Partner: The NHS Feedback Project 186
12.3 Disseminating the Findings of a Corpus-Based Project on Metaphors and Cancer 192
12.4 Conclusion 198

13 Conclusions 201
13.1 Introduction 201

13.2	What Have We Learnt about Health Communication That We Did Not Know Before?	201
13.3	What Advice Would We Pass on to Other Corpus Researchers Working in Health Communication?	203
13.4	What Are the Limitations of the Corpus-Based Approach?	208
13.5	Final Thoughts: What about the Future?	210

Index   *214*

Figures

1.1	Extract from the concordance of the collocational pair *vaccination* and *compulsory*	page 6
2.1	The McGill Pain Questionnaire. (MPQ; Melzack, 1983: 44)	22
3.1	The first page of a transcript document	42
3.2	A passage of the transcript as it appears in the extended context view of CQPweb	45
3.3	Chronological dispersion of texts in the VicVaDis corpus	51
5.1	Response structure for discussion thread 1241	77
7.1	The coefficient of variation	103
7.2	Relative frequencies of words categorised as FOOD over time in UK news articles about obesity	108
9.1	Word Sketch of *anxiety*	137
9.2	Frequencies of Violence metaphors in the corpus per 1,000 words	147

Tables

1.1	Most frequent open-class words in VicVaDis, ordered by raw frequency	*page* 4
1.2	Top-10 open-class collocates of *vaccination* in VicVaDis with a –5/+5 window, ordered by log likelihood	5
1.3	Top-25 keywords from VicVaDis when compared with VicRef, ordered by keyness (likelihood)	7
3.1	Number of articles, words, and mean article lengths in Brookes and Baker's (2021) corpus	36
3.2	Extract of a transcript in the Emergency Department corpus	44
5.1	Forum post metadata for discussion thread 1241	76
5.2	Biber et al.'s (2021) taxonomy for nine communicative purposes	78
5.3	Discourse unit coding for an Opening forum post (Post ID: 1241)	79
5.4	Coding for communicative purposes of discourse units in the thread 1241	81
7.1	Constantly increasing and decreasing high frequency words over time in patient feedback	104
7.2	Monthly keywords for the 'Obesity in the News' corpus	111
7.3	Top-20 keywords (and frequencies) for age groups by decade in the 'Anxiety Forum' corpus	113
7.4	Keywords at various points in the forum posters' journey	115
8.1	Top 25 keywords from VicVaDis when compared with VicRef, ordered by keyness (log likelihood)	123
9.1	Anthropomorphising representation of anxiety	139
9.2	Anxiety as an abstract entity	141
9.3	Word counts in the MELC corpus	145
9.4	Distribution of Violence metaphors in the MELC corpus	147
11.1	Fasce et al.'s (2023) taxonomy of anti-vaccination arguments	172

| 11.2 | Most frequent formulations resulting from the query I ++* (*vac*\|*vax*) | 174 |
| 11.3 | Most frequent formulations resulting from the query I ++* (anti-va*\|antiva*\|anti va*) | 175 |

Acknowledgements

This book is based on research that was funded by the Newby Trust and a series of grants awarded to the authors and their colleagues by UK Research and Innovation (reference numbers ES/K002155/1, ES/R008906/1, ES/J007927/1, ES/V000926/1, and MR/V022954/1).

We are indebted to Andrew Hardie (Lancaster University) for help with data collection and corpus building. We are also grateful to the colleagues and partners who have contributed to our research and its dissemination, including the Institute for Communication in Health Care at the Australian National University, the Hearing the Voice team at Durham University, the project teams for Metaphor in End-of-Life Care and Questioning Vaccination Discourse, and our collaborators at NHS England (Beth Thompson, Ofra Koffman, Clare Enston, and Peter Williamson).

1 Introduction

1.1 Why This Book?

We decided to write this book to document and share the experiences, methods, and findings associated with more than 10 years of corpus linguistic research on health communication in the Department of Linguistics and English Language and the ESRC Centre for Corpus Approaches to Social Science at Lancaster University, UK.

Lancaster University has been at the forefront of the development of corpus linguistics since the 1970s, when expertise in linguistics and computer science began to be combined to create and exploit the large electronic collections of language data known as *corpora* (singular *corpus*, from the Latin word for *body*). Alongside theoretical and empirical contributions to linguistics itself, the Lancaster corpus linguistics tradition has always been focussed on applications of corpus methods beyond linguistics and outside academia. In 2013, this concern for the potential of corpus linguistics to address questions from other disciplines and issues from society at large resulted in the foundation of the Centre for Corpus Approaches to Social Science (CASS), with funding from the Economic and Social Research Council (ESRC, part of UK Research and Innovation). In its first five years, CASS focussed on applications of corpus methods to social science disciplines such as criminology, sociology, and economics, and provided the environment in which our first health-related research blossomed, for example, with projects on metaphors in communication about cancer (Semino et al., 2018) and on patients' online feedback on the National Health Service (NHS) in England (Baker et al., 2019a). Between 2018 and 2024, further ESRC funding for CASS enabled a research programme on health communication specifically, including strands on media representations of obesity (Brookes and Baker, 2021); accounts of lived experience with anxiety, psychosis, and chronic pain (Collins and Baker, 2023; Collins et al., 2023; Semino et al., 2020); and interactions in healthcare settings (Collins et al., 2022). Further funding from ESRC and other sources enabled us to extend our work to discourses around dementia and vaccinations (Brookes, 2023; Coltman-Patel et al., 2022; Putland and Brookes, 2024), and to historical issues such as representations of sexually transmitted diseases in seventeenth-century England (Baker et al., 2019b).

We carried out this work because, alongside linguists working with different methods and in many other universities in the UK and around the world, we believe (and aim to demonstrate that) linguistic expertise has a great deal to offer to research and practices around health and illness (e.g., Demjén, 2020). Much of what we do when we are ill is talk, write, and read about our symptoms, diagnoses, treatment, and outlook. Healthcare professionals communicate with patients and one another as a central part of their jobs. The experiences, causes, and consequences of illness are regular topics of discussion in mainstream media and social media. In this context, a range of linguistic methods and approaches are relevant to understanding the lived experiences of patients, carers, and health professionals; identifying problems and potential solutions in communication in healthcare settings; and investigating public representations of illness and their consequences, especially where prejudice and stigma may be involved. This requires the whole arsenal of theories and methods that linguists have at their disposal, including ethnography, conversation analysis, pragmatics, and, in our case, corpus linguistics (e.g., Brookes and Collins, 2023; Brookes and Hunt, 2021; Demjén, 2020; Hamilton and Chou, 2014; Harvey and Koteyko, 2013).

Corpus methods are particularly relevant where it is possible, necessary, and/or beneficial to collect and study health-related datasets that are too large to be analysed manually. In this book, this usually involves specialised corpora consisting of millions or tens of millions of words, although general corpora can of course be much larger than this. In some cases, large datasets were brought to us by external stakeholders, as in the case of the corpus of NHS feedback discussed in Chapters 2, 6, 11, and 12. In most other cases, we built and analysed corpora from sources where large quantities of data exist and are ethically accessible for research, such as news reports on obesity in Chapters 2, 3, and 10, and online forum posts about cancer in Chapters 5, 9, and 12. While qualitative analyses of small quantities of such data are of course extremely valuable, corpus methods make it possible to combine quantitative information about large-scale patterns with in-depth analyses of specific examples or interactions in context, as also shown in the work by our colleagues in other universities (e.g., Harvey, 2012; Kinloch and Jaworska, 2020; Mullany et al., 2015). Among other things, this in some cases can bridge an unhelpful divide in healthcare research between qualitative and quantitative methods (Greenhalgh, 2016).

Prior to writing this book, we have described the corpora, methods, and findings of our work on health communication in specialised publications (research monographs, articles in linguistic and healthcare journals, specialised edited collections) and in blog posts, podcasts, and media interviews for the general public. Through this book, we aim to present our work, and what can be learnt from it, for the benefit of readers who are not already experts in corpus linguistics, healthcare research, or either. This includes students and, more generally, anyone who might seek guidance or inspiration in beginning to use corpus methods to study health communication or beginning to apply their expertise in corpus methods to health communication. To achieve this, we have not simply endeavoured to present our work in a more accessible way than in more specialised writing, but we have included details about aspects of the research that are not suitable for other forms of publication, such as different ways of formulating research questions, dealing with ethical issues, and engaging with non-academic stakeholders. In this way, we hope to make our experiences over the last 10 years as useful to our readers as we can.

It is beyond the scope of this book to provide a detailed introduction to corpus linguistics and the different tools and techniques associated with it. Several such introductions already exist, such as McEnery and Hardie (2011), O'Keeffe and McCarthy (2021), and Hunston (2022). Nonetheless, in the next section we provide a brief overview of the main corpus linguistic techniques that are referred to in the rest of the book, for the benefit of readers unfamiliar with corpus linguistics.

1.2 An Overview of Corpus Linguistic Analytical Techniques

Corpus linguistics, as we have mentioned, involves the use of tailor-made software tools to study patterns of linguistic choices in digital collections of texts, or corpora, that are too large to analyse by hand or eye alone (McEnery and Hardie, 2011). Such software tools make it possible, among other things, to study the frequencies of words, patterns of co-occurrence of words (collocations), instances of words in context (concordances), and unusually frequent words (keywords). In fact, corpus tools make it possible to carry out the same analyses at the level of grammatical categories and semantic fields. In this section, however, we will demonstrate the technique at the level of words.

More specifically, we will briefly demonstrate each of these techniques with reference to a three-million-word corpus of literature (mainly pamphlets) from the Victorian period in England that opposed vaccination against smallpox, which was made compulsory in 1853: the Victorian Anti-Vaccination Discourse corpus (VicVaDis). The composition of the corpus is described in detail in Chapter 3, and an example of exploitation of the corpus is provided in Chapter 8, based on Hardaker and colleagues (2024). The analyses carried out were obtained by loading texts into the free corpus analysis tool AntConc (Anthony, 2022; www.laurenceanthony.net/software/antconc/). Many other tools are available, and several will be mentioned in the course of this book, including CQPweb (Hardie, 2012; https://cqpweb.lancs.ac.uk),

Sketch Engine (Kilgarriff et al., 2014; www.sketchengine.eu), Wmatrix (Rayson, 2008; https://ucrel-wmatrix6.lancaster.ac.uk/wmatrix6.html), and WordSmith Tools (Scott, 2016; www.lexically.net/wordsmith/). Each offers a range of similar functions, along with some which are unique. It is beyond the scope of this book to provide introductions to these different corpus tools, but in all cases online guides or tutorials are available for both novice and advanced users.

1.2.1 Frequency Lists

An initial exploration of a corpus may involve the extraction of a frequency list – namely, a list of all the words included in the corpus, in decreasing order of frequency. The topmost frequent words in a corpus tend to be grammatical words, such as (in English) *the*, *of*, and *it*. To begin to explore the VicVaDis corpus, Hardaker and colleagues (2024) extract a frequency list of lexical, or open-class, words (i.e., nouns, verbs, adjectives, and adverbs). They then present the top 10 most frequent lexical words in the corpus (Table 1.1; note that in the final row, *jenner* references the surname of the doctor who is credited with the introduction of vaccination against smallpox in England). Table 1.1 includes both the raw frequencies and the relative or normalised frequencies per million words. Normalised frequencies are particularly relevant when comparing corpora of different sizes.

Hardaker and colleagues (2024) begin by studying the use of the most frequent lexical word in the VicVaDis corpus (i.e., the noun *vaccination*).

Table 1.1 *Most frequent open-class words in VicVaDis, ordered by raw frequency*

Word	Raw frequency	Normalised frequency per million words
vaccination	31,734	9,095.55
smallpox	21,874	6,269.492
dr	11,186	3,206.114
mr	9,608	2,753.83
vaccinated	8,876	2,544.025
disease	8,592	2,462.626
medical	7,793	2,233.618
years	7,150	2,049.322
cases	6,258	1,793.658
jenner	5,345	1,531.976

Adapted from Hardaker et al. (2024): 168.

1.2 An Overview of Corpus Linguistic Analytical Techniques

Table 1.2 *Top-10 open-class collocates of* vaccination *in VicVaDis with a –5/+ 5 window, ordered by log likelihood*

Collocate	Frequency	Likelihood	Effect
compulsory	2,223	5,583.747	3.032
after	1,350	1,255.124	1.639
question	1,048	1,181.757	1.839
inquirer	379	1,053.572	3.243
anti	769	991.075	1.994
acts	453	947.557	2.697
against	1,055	846.510	1.504
act	694	749.524	1.793
league	251	532.783	2.723
tracts	184	474.361	3.087

Adapted from Hardaker et al. (2024): 169.

1.2.2 Collocates

One way of understanding how particular words are used in a corpus is to look at what other words tend to occur around them more frequently than one would expect by chance. Such words are known as the *collocates* of that particular word of interest, or *node* word. Patterns of collocation can reveal the meanings and associations of words in a particular corpus.

Hardaker and colleagues (2024) extract from the VicVaDis corpus the collocates of the noun *vaccination* – the most frequent open-class word. Table 1.2 provides the top 10 open-class collocates of *vaccination*. They were identified within a window of five words to the left and five words to the right of the node word, and by means of two statistical measures: a measure of statistical significance, log likelihood, which captures the probability that the relationship between two words may occur by chance (see the 'Likelihood' column); and a measure of effect size, which captures the strength of the collocation between the node word and each collocate. The table also provides the overall number of occurrences of the collocational pair in the corpus (see the 'Frequency' column).

Hardaker and colleagues (2024) then focus on the collocation between *compulsory* and *vaccination*, to identify objections to the mandatory nature of the smallpox vaccine in the VicVaDis corpus.

1.2.3 Concordances

A more detailed, qualitative way of studying the use of particular words or combinations of words in a corpus is to obtain a *concordance* (i.e., all instances of that word or combination of words in context). Figure 1.1

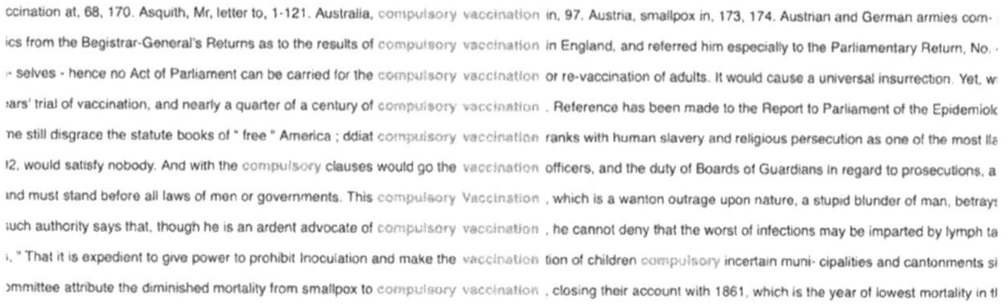

1 Introduction

[concordance extract]

ccination at, 68, 170. Asquith, Mr, letter to, 1-121. Australia, compulsory vaccination in, 97. Austria, smallpox in, 173, 174. Austrian and German armies com-
ics from the Begistrar-General's Returns as to the results of compulsory vaccination in England, and referred him especially to the Parliamentary Return, No.
selves - hence no Act of Parliament can be carried for the compulsory vaccination or re-vaccination of adults. It would cause a universal insurrection. Yet, w
ars' trial of vaccination, and nearly a quarter of a century of compulsory vaccination . Reference has been made to the Report to Parliament of the Epidemiol
ne still disgrace the statute books of " free " America ; ddiat compulsory vaccination ranks with human slavery and religious persecution as one of the most ll
l2, would satisfy nobody. And with the compulsory clauses would go the vaccination officers, and the duty of Boards of Guardians in regard to prosecutions, a
nd must stand before all laws of men or governments. This compulsory vaccination , which is a wanton outrage upon nature, a stupid blunder of man, betray:
uch authority says that, though he is an ardent advocate of compulsory vaccination , he cannot deny that the worst of infections may be imparted by lymph ta
i, " That it is expedient to give power to prohibit Inoculation and make the vaccination tion of children compulsory incertain muni- cipalities and cantonments si
ommittee attribute the diminished mortality from smallpox to compulsory vaccination , closing their account with 1861, which is the year of lowest mortality in tl

Figure 1.1 Extract from the concordance of the collocational pair *vaccination* and *compulsory*.

provides an extract from the concordance of *compulsory* collocating with *vaccination* in the VicVaDis corpus.

Hardaker and colleagues (2024) explore the concordance to identify the main objections to compulsory vaccination in the corpus, such as, for example, that it is unnatural and a violation of civil liberties.

1.2.4 Keywords

Finally, *keyness* analysis makes it possible to identify the distinctive vocabulary in a corpus of interest (the 'target' corpus) by comparing the relative or normalised frequencies of words against a corpus that can be seen as a relevant norm (the 'reference' corpus). The resulting 'keywords' are words that are statistically 'overused' in the target corpus as compared with the reference corpus.

Hardaker and colleagues (2024) extract the keywords in the VicVaDis corpus by comparing it against a reference corpus labelled the VicRef corpus (see Chapter 8 for more detail). The reference corpus consists of a tailor-made nineteenth-century corpus containing texts from similar genres but involving a wide variety of topics. The top 25 keywords are presented in Table 1.3. The table includes raw and normalised frequencies for both corpora, as well as scores for the same two statistical measures we have mentioned in the section on collocations.

In corpus analyses, keywords are often grouped according to particular themes, based on semantic similarity, grammatical similarity, or a combination of the two. Subsequently, selected groups are subjected to more detailed analysis. For example, as we show in Chapter 8, Hardaker and colleagues (2024) look at concordance lines for the keywords *death*, *deaths*, *disease*, and *diseases* as a grouping of semantically related terms in order to identify the different kinds of harms that are attributed to vaccination, and the ways in which those harms are presented.

Table 1.3 Top-25 keywords from VicVaDis when compared with VicRef, ordered by keyness (likelihood)

Rank	Type	Raw frequency: VicVaDis	Raw frequency: VicRef	Normalised frequency per million words: VicVaDis	Normalised frequency per million words: VicRef	Keyness (likelihood)	Keyness (effect)
1	vaccination	31,734	4	9,095.55	2.005	28,736.667	0.018
2	smallpox	21,874	4	6,269.492	2.005	19,765.969	0.012
3	vaccinated	8,876	3	2,544.025	1.504	7,988.536	0.005
4	disease	8,592	116	2,462.626	58.142	6,780.952	0.005
5	dr	11,186	636	3,206.114	318.781	6,459.756	0.006
6	Medical	7,793	64	2,233.618	32.079	6,441.045	0.004
7	jenner	5,345	0	1,531.976	0	4,837.453	0.003
8	cowpox	4,687	0	1,343.381	0	4,241.613	0.003
9	mr	9,608	1,140	2,753.83	571.399	3,731.588	0.005
10	lymph	3,586	5	1,027.814	2.506	3,179.169	0.002
11	was	29,005	8,671	8,313.368	4,346.144	3,141.183	0.016
12	vaccine	3,517	8	1,008.037	4.01	3,085.139	0.002
13	inoculation	3,416	3	979.089	1.504	3,048.773	0.002
14	deaths	3,441	28	986.254	14.034	2,844.497	0.002
15	mortality	3,373	34	966.764	17.042	2,739.78	0.002
16	compulsory	2,989	14	856.703	7.017	2,554.487	0.002
17	epidemic	2,867	9	821.735	4.511	2,490.431	0.002
18	years	7,150	997	2,049.322	499.724	2,430.964	0.004
19	diseases	3,059	40	876.766	20.049	2,421.166	0.002
20	unvaccinated	2,184	0	625.975	0	1,975.893	0.001
21	cases	6,258	962	1,793.658	482.181	1,940.183	0.004
22	cannot	2,116	0	606.485	0	1,914.357	0.001
23	london	4,198	443	1,203.224	222.044	1,770.514	0.002
24	hospital	2,276	36	652.344	18.044	1,760.796	0.001
25	death	3,739	335	1,071.666	167.911	1,744.884	0.002

1.3 The Structure of This Book

In this book we demonstrate the kinds of questions, settings, and datasets that can be involved in corpus-based studies of health communication, and the variety of tools that can be employed to carry out these studies. We aim to do this in a way that is maximally useful to readers who are not already experts in this area, and especially students. Thus, we have structured the chapters according to the likely sequential stages of the research process: from research questions to dissemination, with some chapters on selected topics for analysis in the middle. Each chapter demonstrates the relevant stage of research or topic with reference to two or three specific projects that at least one of us has been involved with at Lancaster University. While all five co-authors take responsibility for the whole book, in this section we indicate who is particularly responsible for each chapter. In the chapter itself, we also mention team members not involved in this book, where relevant.

Following the present introductory chapter (by Semino), Chapter 2 (by Baker and Semino) is devoted to the formulation of research questions. We discuss the different processes through which research questions can be identified and developed in corpus-based research on health communication, depending on the nature of the project and the degree of involvement of different stakeholders. Three studies are considered, in order to compare how various research questions were formulated. The first study involved the analysis of press representations of obesity (Brookes and Baker, 2021). In this study, the researchers developed their own research questions in a variety of ways, including, for example, by drawing from the non-linguistic literature on obesity. The second study focussed on the McGill Pain Questionnaire (MPQ) – a well-known language-based diagnostic tool for pain. A pain consultant asked the researchers if they could help understand why some patients find it difficult to respond to some sections of the questionnaire. In response, the researchers formulated a series of questions that could be answered using corpus linguistic tools and identified some issues with the questionnaire that address the pain consultant's concerns (Semino et al., 2020). The third study (Baker et al., 2019a) involved the analysis of patient feedback on the NHS. The researchers were approached by the NHS Feedback Team and given 12 questions that they were commissioned to answer by means of corpus linguistic methods.

In Chapter 3 (by Brookes, Collins, and Semino), we reflect on different approaches to data collection, drawing on our own experiences of corpus creation to highlight the opportunities and challenges associated with building corpora from health communication data. We begin with a case study based on a purpose-built corpus of news articles on the topic of obesity, collected from the LexisNexis online news repository. We focus on theoretical considerations attending to corpus design (i.e., the 'aboutness' of the

1.3 The Structure of This Book

texts collected and the balance and representativeness of the corpus as a whole), as well as practical challenges involved in processing texts provided by repositories such as LexisNexis to make them amenable to corpus analysis (e.g., removing repeated texts, noise, boilerplate text, etc.). The second case study focusses on how corpus linguists might work with existing datasets of health communication data – in this case, transcripts collected by research collaborators conducting ethnographic research in the context of Australian emergency departments. We discuss the ways in which data collected by researchers for the purposes of different kinds of analysis is likely to require some pre-processing before we can consider it a corpus suitable for corpus-based analysis. The third case study is concerned with the creation of the VicVaDis corpus, which we mentioned earlier. We discuss the challenges and decisions involved in sourcing historical material from existing databases, selecting a principled set of potential candidate texts for inclusion and using optical character recognition (OCR) software to convert the texts into a format that is appropriate for the use of corpus tools.

In Chapter 4 (by Semino and Brookes), we consider ethical issues in healthcare communication research through two case studies. The first case study looks at a relatively straightforward situation involving a study of the Pain Concern online forum. Data from the forum was provided by HealthUnlocked, a company that runs a large number of online communities related to health. One advantage of using their service was that HealthUnlocked took care of relevant legal requirements concerning ethics and only shared data from contributors to the forum who had agreed for their posts to be used for research purposes. The second case study relates to the study of dementia and brings into focus the difficulties of working with multiple datasets and a range of stakeholders. The data collection for this project involved public health communication in terms of news media and external communications from support services, including social media. As such, it presents scenarios that are common to studies of health communication and thereby offers instruction in how to navigate related ethical concerns.

In Chapter 5 (by Collins and Semino), we are concerned with documenting and investigating sequential aspects of health-oriented interactions and the particular challenges this poses for corpus-based research. We describe two case studies to demonstrate how conventional corpus procedures can be augmented with other linguistic approaches to facilitate a critical examination of the meaningful relationships between parts of the data that might otherwise be separated in corpus analysis, as individual texts or as participant turns in a discussion, for example. The first case study involves an approach that was developed through an investigation of the Spoken British National Corpus (BNC) 2014 to examine interactional language texts in terms of functional discourse units (Biber et al., 2021; Egbert et al., 2021). This coding framework is applied to a sample of anxiety support forum data in order to document, quantify, and evaluate how various communicative purposes are formulated in forum posts and are met with different types of response. The second case study is an investigation of a specific discussion thread from an online forum dedicated to cancer – one that is explicitly dedicated to irreverent verbal play about the illness. We show how a corpus approach enabled the identification of relevant humorous metaphors and made it possible to identify recurrent lexical and grammatical features that serve important functions for facilitating discussion around sensitive topics, maintaining a coherent identity and contributing to a sense of community.

In Chapter 6 (by Brookes), we turn to how it is possible to use demographic metadata to study identities in health-related corpora. We employ two case studies to demonstrate and compare two broad approaches to identifying and studying demographic characteristics, based on research on patient feedback on NHS services in England. The first case study compares how patients of different age and sex groups evaluate healthcare services and, more specifically, how they use distinct linguistic and rhetorical strategies to do this (see Baker et al., 2019a). The corpus was encoded with demographic metadata which allowed the researchers to explore the language used by people of different age and sex identity groups when evaluating the care and treatment they received for cancer (see Brookes and Baker, 2022). For the second study, a different corpus of more general patient feedback was used, one which did not contain demographic information metadata about patients' identities. Instead, targeted searches were used to identify patients' demographic characteristics based on cases where they made those characteristics explicit within their feedback (e.g., through statements like 'I am a 55-year-old woman'). In contrasting these case studies, we also evaluate the two different approaches taken, considering the affordances and limitations of both. Taken together, the case studies demonstrate how language and identity can be explored in corpora with and without reliable demographic metadata.

In Chapter 7 (by Baker), we consider how language changes over short time spans can be examined using corpus-assisted methods. We present three case studies which consider time in different ways. The first involves the corpus of patient feedback relating to cancer care, as described in Chapter 6. This data had been collected for four consecutive years, so to compare change over time, a technique called the coefficient of variation was used to identify lexical items that had increased or decreased over time. These items were examined through concordance lines in order to uncover some of the strongest trends in terms of patient satisfaction. The second case study considered UK newspaper articles about obesity, ranging from 2008 to 2017. To examine changing themes over time, a combination of keyness and concordance analyses was employed in order to identify which themes in the corpus were becoming more or less popular over

1.3 The Structure of This Book

time. We show how references to individual causes of obesity (e.g., diet or biological determinants) had become more popular over the years, whereas societal causes (e.g., the role of education, government, advertising, or businesses) had decreased. Additionally, the analysis considered time in a different way, by using the concept of the annual news cycle. To this end, the corpus was divided into 12 parts, consisting of articles published according to a particular month, and the same type of analysis was applied to each part. Annual patterns were found around the reporting of obesity (e.g., readers were advised to join a gym in January, whereas sleep and yoga were suggested as weight loss options in February). The third case study involves an analysis of a corpus of forum posts about anxiety from 2012 to 2020. In this study, time was considered in terms of the age of the poster. Younger posters tended to use more catastrophising language and help-seeking posts, whereas older posters tended to offer different forms of advice, which became increasingly less focussed around medical intervention, the older they were. However, time was also considered in terms of the amount of involvement that a poster had with the forum. It was found that posters progressed from initially seeking advice and providing their personal histories to increasingly taking on an emotionally supportive or advice-giving role. The more experienced posters characterised their relationship with anxiety as a learning experience or journey.

In Chapter 8 (by McEnery and Semino), we look are combined at the use of historical corpora in the study of language relating to health. We present two case studies – one where an issue is well understood and discussed publicly, the other where there was a clear issue with the framing of a discussion. The first case study explores the VicVaDis corpus, briefly introduced earlier in this chapter. Different corpus techniques to show the main anti-vaccination arguments in the corpus and to point out parallels with present-day anti-vaccination discourse. The second case study looks at the emergence of venereal disease in the seventeenth century using the Early English Books Online corpus. We show how, by examining the collocates of the word *pox*, it is possible to identify relevant uses of the word (e.g., those which referred to venereal disease as opposed to those which do not). Additionally, we show that through the investigation of one type of collocate (words referring to geographical locations), the analysis was taken in an unexpected but rewarding direction.

Chapter 9 (by Baker and Semino) considers how the experience of illness is represented linguistically, focussing on two contexts. In the first case study, collocational patterns were examined in order to show how people represented the word *anxiety*. Different patterns around anxiety were grouped together in order to identify oppositional pairs of representation (e.g., medicalising/normalising). The second case study involved an examination of the ways in which cancer was constructed in a corpus of interviews with and online forum posts by people with cancer, family carers, and healthcare professionals. Using a combination of manual analysis and corpus searches, it was possible to consider how metaphors were used to convey a sense of empowerment or disempowerment in the experience of cancer. More specifically, the analysis of metaphors around cancer revealed insights into people's identity construction and the relationships between doctors and patients.

In Chapter 10 (by Baker and Collins), we demonstrate how corpus approaches support the study of various social actors, which in the healthcare context can include healthcare professionals, patients, caregivers, and even manifestations of illness. Our first case study investigates how representations of people with obesity in the UK press contribute to stigmatisation. The analysis orients around the naming strategies to collectively and individually refer to people with obesity, as well as the adjectives used to describe them and the activities that they are reported to be involved in. For example, we demonstrate a high degree of shaming in the UK press using informal, dehumanising labels such as 'fatties', 'lardy', and 'blob'. Furthermore, we show that people with obesity are regularly held up as figures of ridicule and obesity is discussed in the context of social deviance, foregrounded when reporting on perpetrators of crimes. In the second case study, we similarly discuss referential strategies, descriptions of traits, and the capacity to carry out different kinds of actions in the context of voice-hearing, to critically consider the different degrees to which people who experience psychosis personify their voices. To facilitate this analysis, it was necessary to develop a means of corpus annotation and adapt procedures for quantifying linguistic features that we argue can be more generally applied to investigations of social actors. We discuss how this corpus approach enables researchers and other stakeholders to track these representations in the reports of those with lived experience over time and consider the implications of a social actor model for therapeutic interventions to support those with chronic mental health issues.

Chapter 11 (by Brookes, Collins, and Semino) introduces the concept of legitimation in discourse and considers how it might function and be studied in the context of health(care) communication. First, we look at how contributors to the online parenting forum Mumsnet use labels denoting attitudes towards vaccinations, such as 'pro-vax' and 'anti-vax'. We point out how labels that involve opposition to vaccinations, such as 'anti-vaxxer', tend to collocate with negation, and then consider in detail how people justify negating the applicability of the label to themselves. This reveals a range of different concerns around vaccinations. We then draw on a case study of patient feedback (see also Chapter 6) which examined how patients legitimate their perspectives and the evaluations they gave in their feedback. For example, this included patients representing themselves as experienced users of healthcare services (or 'expert patients'). Additionally, some patients used aspects of their identities in order to position themselves as requiring attention, while others engaged in linguistic

1.3 The Structure of This Book

techniques such as second-person pronouns to imply that their experiences could be generalised to other patients. Overall, the chapter underscores the need for close, qualitative examination of words and wider linguistic devices within their broader textual and health(care) contexts in order to interpret the legitimatory functions of given linguistic patterns.

Chapter 12 (by Baker and Semino) discusses the potential opportunities and challenges associated with disseminating the findings of corpus-based approaches to health communication, which also apply more generally to interdisciplinary research and collaborations between researchers and non-academic stakeholders. The first case study involves work on patient feedback with members of the NHS who had provided a list of questions for us to work on. We discuss the importance of and challenges around building and maintaining relationships with members of this large, changing organisation, while also outlining how we approached the dissemination of findings, both in academic and non-academic senses, and the extent of our impact. The second case study considers the experience of disseminating findings from the project on metaphors and cancer introduced in Chapter 5, focussing particularly on writing for a healthcare journal, dealing with the media, and going beyond corpus data to create a metaphor-based resource for communication about cancer.

Chapter 13 (by Baker) concludes the book by presenting a synthesis of the previous chapters, beginning by asking the question, 'What have our experiences taught us about health communication that we didn't know?' We go on to examine lessons we learnt about carrying out corpus-based research on health communication, offering practical advice and tips for people who might be carrying out similar kinds of studies. We then consider the limitations of a corpus-based approach and end by looking to the future: what changes have taken place since we completed our analyses? What kinds of developments in the field of healthcare and in corpus linguistic analysis have occurred recently? And what avenues of research into health care do we believe are potentially interesting to investigate next?

We hope that this book will enable and inspire readers to pursue their own investigations, going beyond what we and others have achieved so far.

References

Anthony, L. (2022). AntConc (Version 4.2.0) [Computer Software]. Waseda University. Available from www.laurenceanthony.net/software.

Baker, P., Brookes, G. and Evans, C. (2019a). *The Language of Patient Feedback: A Corpus Linguistic Study of Online Health Communication*. Routledge.

Baker, H., Gregory, I., Hartmann, D. and McEnery, T. (2019b). Applying Geographical Information Systems to Researching Historical Corpora: Seventeenth Century

Prostitution. In V. Wiegand and M. Mahlberg (eds.), *Corpus Linguistics, Context and Culture* (pp. 109–36). De Gruyter.

Biber, D., Egbert, J., Keller, D. and Wizner, S. (2021). Towards a Taxonomy of Conversational Discourse Types: An Empirical Corpus-Based Analysis. *Journal of Pragmatics*, *171*, 20–35. https://doi.org/10.1016/j.pragma.2020.09.018.

Brookes, G. (2023). Killer, Thief or Companion? A Corpus-Based Study of Dementia Metaphors in UK Tabloids. *Metaphor and Symbol*, *38*(3), 213–30. https://doi.org/10.1080/10926488.2022.2142472.

Brookes, G. and Baker, P. (2021). *Obesity in the News: Language and Representation in the British Press*. Cambridge University Press.

Brookes, G. and Collins, L. (2023). *Corpus Linguistics for Health Communication: A Guide for Research*. Routledge.

Brookes, G. and Hunt, D. (2021). *Analysing Health Communication: Discourse Approaches*. Palgrave Macmillan.

Collins, L. C. and Baker, P. (2023) *Language, Discourse and Anxiety*. Cambridge University Press.

Collins, L. C., Brezina, V., Demjén, Z., Semino, E. and Woods, A. (2023). Corpus Linguistics and Clinical Psychology: Investigating Personification in First-Person Accounts of Voice-Hearing. *International Journal of Corpus Linguistics*, *28*(1), 28–59. https://doi.org/10.1075/ijcl.21019.col.

Collins, L. C., Gablasova, D. and Pill, J. (2022). 'Doing Questioning' in the Emergency Department (ED). *Health Communication*. Online first. 1–9. https://doi.org/10.1080/10410236.2022.2111630.

Coltman-Patel, T., Dance, W., Demjén, Z., Gatherer, D., Hardaker, C. and Semino, E. (2022). Am I Being Unreasonable to Vaccinate My Kids against My Ex's Wishes?' – A Corpus Linguistic Exploration of Conflict in Vaccination Discussions on Mumsnet Talk's AIBU Forum. *Discourse, Context & Media*, *48*, 100624. https://doi.org/10.1016/j.dcm.2022.100624.

Demjén, Z. (ed.) (2020). *Applying Linguistics in Illness and Healthcare Contexts*. Bloomsbury.

Egbert, J., Wizner, S., Keller, D., Biber, D., McEnery, T. and Baker, P. (2021). Identifying and Describing Functional Discourse Units in the BNC Spoken 2014. *Text & Talk*, *41*(5–6), 715–37. https://doi.org/10.1515/text-2020-0053.

Greenhalgh T. (2016). *Cultural Contexts of Health: The Use of Narrative Research in the Health Sector*. Copenhagen: WHO Regional Office for Europe. https://iris.who.int/handle/10665/326310.

Hardie, A. (2012). CQPweb – Combining Power, Flexibility and Usability in a Corpus Analysis Tool. *International Journal of Corpus Linguistics*, *17*(3), 380–409. https://doi.org/10.1075/ijcl.17.3.04har.

Kinloch, K. and Jaworska, S. (2020). Using a Comparative Corpus-Assisted Approach to Study Health and Illness Discourses across Domains: The Case of Postnatal Depression (PND) in Lay, Medical and Media Texts. In Z. Demjén (ed.), *Applying Linguistics in Illness and Healthcare Contexts* (pp. 73–98). Bloomsbury.

Hamilton, H. and Chou, W. S. (eds.) (2014). *The Routledge Handbook of Language and Health Communication*. Routledge.

Hardaker, C., Deignan, A., Semino, E., Coltman-Patel, T., Dance, W., Demjén, Z., Sanderson, C. and Gatherer, D. (2024). The Victorian Anti-Vaccination Discourse

1.3 The Structure of This Book

Corpus (VicVaDis): Construction and Exploration. *Digital Scholarship in the Humanities*, *39*, 162–74. https://doi.org/10.1093/llc/fqad075.
Harvey, K. (2012). Disclosures of Depression: Using Corpus Linguistics Methods to Examine Young People's Online Health Concerns. *International Journal of Corpus Linguistics*, *17*(3), 349–79. https://doi.org/10.1075/ijcl.17.3.03har.
Harvey, K. and Koteyko, N. (2013). *Exploring Health Communication: Language in Action*. Routledge.
Hunston, S. (2022). *Corpora in Applied Linguistics*, 2nd ed. Cambridge University Press.
Kilgarriff, A., Baisa, V., Bušta, J., Jakubíček, M., Kovář, V., Michelfeit, J., Rychlý, P. and Suchomel, V. (2014). The Sketch Engine: Ten Years On. *Lexicography*, *1*, 7–36. https://doi.org/10.1007/s40607-014-0009-9.
McEnery, T. and Hardie, A. (2011). *Corpus Linguistics: Method, Theory and Practice*. Cambridge University Press.
Mullany, L., Smith, C., Harvey, K. and Adolphs, S. (2015). 'Am I Anorexic?' Weight, Eating and Discourses of the Body in Online Adolescent Health Communication. *Communication & Medicine*, *12*(2–3), 211–23. https://doi.org/10.1558/cam.16692.
O'Keeffe, A. and McCarthy, M. J. (2021). *The Routledge Handbook of Corpus Linguistics*, 2nd ed. Routledge.
Putland, E. and Brookes, G. (2024) Dementia Stigma: Representation and Language Use. *Journal of Language and Aging Research*, *2*(1), 5–46. https://doi.org/10.15460/jlar.2024.2.1.1266.
Rayson, P. (2008). From Key Words to Key Semantic Domains. *International Journal of Corpus Linguistics*, *13*(4), 519–49. https://doi.org/10.1075/ijcl.13.4.06ray.
Scott, M. (2016). *WordSmith Tools* (Version 7). Lexical Analysis Software.
Semino, E., Demjén, Z., Hardie, A., Payne, S. and Rayson, P. (2018). *Metaphor, Cancer and the End of Life: A Corpus-Based Study*. Routledge.
Semino, E., Hardie, A. and Zakzrewska, J. M. (2020). Applying Corpus Linguistics to a Diagnostic Tool for Pain. In Z. Demjén (ed.), *Applying Linguistics in Illness and Healthcare Contexts* (pp. 99–128). Bloomsbury.

2 Research Questions

2.1 Introduction

Research projects generally involve the formulation of questions that researchers aim to answer via the most appropriate combination of data and methods. In many disciplines, research questions are a requirement in students' dissertation/thesis proposals and in researchers' applications for funding. In practice, research projects do not always begin with specific questions, and even when they do, those questions often evolve over time. However, the development of research questions tends to happen early in the research process, which is why we consider this topic here in this second chapter.

Broadly speaking, research questions need to be relevant and viable in the context where they are intended to be answered. However, exactly what counts as an appropriate research question varies from discipline to discipline and context to context. With regard to projects in linguistics, Sunderland (2010) and Wray and Bloomer (2021) provide useful reflections and guidance. In this chapter we draw from our experience to focus more specifically on the different ways research questions can be developed in corpus-based studies of health communication. We have selected three case studies that contrast with each other in terms of when and how research questions were formulated and how much control we as linguists had in that process.

The first case study involves the analysis of a corpus of UK news articles about obesity. Here the researchers had a considerable degree of freedom in how to approach the study and, specifically, in terms of when and how to formulate research questions. We show how the researchers began with an initial exploratory approach to the data by means of a keyness analysis. They then went on to develop goals and priorities for the research in an organic, cyclical manner that also involved literature reviews and interactions with stakeholders. By these methods, they arrived at a set of specific research aims which, for some purposes, were expressed as a series of research questions.

The second case study involves the exploitation of an existing corpus of English to investigate potential weaknesses in the language used in a diagnostic questionnaire for pain. Here the linguists involved in the research were approached by a pain clinician who wanted to know why her patients seemed to have difficulties with some specific aspects of the pain questionnaire. The researchers then turned the clinician's broad question into a series of specific research questions that could be answered by means of corpus linguistic methods. We show how this made it possible to identify some aspects of the language used in the questionnaire that explained the difficulties observed by the clinician and that also had wider relevance for any health professional using the questionnaire.

The third case study involves the analysis of a corpus of patients' online feedback on the services of the National Health Service (NHS) in England. Here the linguists involved in the research were approached by NHS England and provided with a set of 12 pre-formulated questions that the researchers had to answer in a very tight timeframe. We show how the researchers answered these questions by creatively and eclectically employing the corpus linguistic tools most appropriate for each question. We also point out how some of the original questions had to be adapted in interaction with the external partners and how some additional questions were formulated in response to initial findings. Eventually, all 12 preset questions were answered to the satisfaction of NHS England and within the required timeframe.

Throughout this chapter, we discuss both the challenges and the opportunities associated with each of these different approaches to the development of research questions.

2.2 Developing Exploratory Questions

Perhaps one of the most common ways of approaching a corpus-assisted discourse analysis project is to develop and refine questions as a result of exploratory analyses in a bottom-up manner, an approach which draws on grounded theory (Glaser and Strauss, 1967). Rather than beginning with a specific set of questions, the analyst approaches the corpus in a reasonably naïve and open way, simply asking 'What is interesting, (unexpectedly) frequent, or unusual in this corpus?' and letting the initial answers to those questions lead to further questions. To illustrate this approach, we describe a study (Brookes and Baker, 2021) which involved the analysis of a 36-million-word corpus of newspaper articles about obesity published between 2008 and 2017, with articles drawn from 11 national UK newspapers. Brookes and Baker chose to carry out this analysis by engaging with existing (non-corpus) research which had highlighted problematic aspects of news reporting around obesity; they also drew from their own hypothesis, based on analysing a smaller sample of data, that a corpus approach would be fruitful. They did not begin with any specific lists of words or other linguistic phenomena which they wanted to examine, although they decided to devise a set of possible ways to approach the analysis.

One approach was to apply some form of comparative analysis. As the corpus contained articles from 11 newspapers across 10 years, 2 obvious forms of analysis were selected. The first was a comparison across newspapers. Based on a previous comparative approach to a corpus of articles about Islam (Baker et al., 2013), Brookes and Baker (2021) decided that making distinctions between 11 newspapers would not be appropriate, especially because some newspapers contributed much smaller amounts of corpus data than others. Instead, they carried out a four-way comparison, based on the tabloid versus broadsheet formats and left versus right political perspectives. They grouped the *Express*, *Mail*, *Star*, and *Sun* into right-leaning tabloids, while the *Guardian*, *Independent*, and *i Paper* were considered together as left-leaning broadsheets. Keyword comparisons between these sets of newspapers highlighted the major lexical differences and similarities among them. Additionally, the researchers considered cases where a single newspaper contributed towards the majority of instances of a specific keyword.

As the corpus consisted of a decade of articles, Brookes and Baker also considered change over time, taking each year of data separately and tracking lexical changes over time. This enabled them to identify how the newspapers gradually moved towards emphasising personal responsibility and biological frames around obesity, while de-emphasising the societal frame. They also took a different perspective on change over time (see Chapter 7) by considering the annual news cycle consisting of 12 months. They then compared the articles published in January (across all years) against articles from February and so on. This approach was inspired by Anna Marchi's PhD research, which looked at a single year of the *Guardian*. In her thesis she writes:

> Firstly it should be noted that there is no particularly good reason to choose a calendar year as unit, but it is purely a matter of cultural habit: most societies, in fact, regulate their existence and its interpretation following what Bettini calls 'the power of the calendar' (1995: 21, my translation). A year span was therefore chosen for reasons of convention and the span was limited to one complete and continuous year of the newspaper's life, in order to limit the impact of the diachronic variable. (Marchi, 2014: 15)

The analysis carried out by Brookes and Baker which compared months was able to show how stories about obesity operate in a repetitive annual cycle, with different topics and discourses occurring at various points throughout the year. For example, in January there was a focus on starting a new diet and joining a gym, whereas during the summer months there were articles relaying concerns about being seen in swimwear while on holiday.

Another aspect of the analysis was inspired by the researchers' engagement with non-linguistic literature on obesity, particularly published work around gender, health, and the body (e.g., Bordo, 1993; Gill et al., 2000; Gough, 2010).

2.2 Developing Exploratory Questions

Other aspects were inspired by conversations with experts from other disciplines and stakeholders, where researchers were encouraged to view discourses around obesity through a lens of social class. This led them to carry out analyses which focussed on different kinds of social actor representation in the corpus of articles: men and women, as well as the terms *under-class*, *working class*, *middle class*, and *upper class*.

By engaging with these initial comparative studies, the analysis helped identify other aspects within the corpus which felt ripe for more detailed study. One of these was the presence of shaming and stigmatising language, which had been identified at an early stage in the research as appearing more clearly in the right-leaning tabloids (e.g., through noun labels like *fatty* and *hog*, adjectives like *lardy* or *blobby*, or verbs like *guzzle* and *waddle*), although more subtle uses of stigmatising language had also been identified in broadsheet newspapers (e.g., the nomination *the obese*). Although stigma was not too frequent in the news, it felt like a salient theme and also one of the most problematic aspects of the articles, from a critical perspective. Therefore, this was deemed worthy of a separate analysis, which Chapter 10 of this book describes in detail. Generally, the phenomenon of stigmatising language has been of particular interest to charities and other groups outside academia.

Finally, the researchers decided to focus part of the analysis around four specific words which they had identified as highly frequent or having a high keyness score in the corpus, as well as collocating with one another. These words were *healthy*, *body*, *diet*, and *exercise*. All four words were significant in that they were used in articles which focussed on different ways of reducing obesity, although they were also used in a wide range of ways, indicating that different meanings and discourses were realised through them.

It is notable that throughout the monograph based on the analysis of this corpus (Brookes and Baker, 2021), there is only one explicit mention of 'research questions', and there is no place in the book where all the research questions are listed, as in Baker and colleagues' (2019) book on NHS feedback, described later in this chapter. Instead, at the start of each chapter of the book, the researchers outlined the topic they aimed to *explore* (e.g., forms of this verb occur 35 times across the book, and it is a word used particularly often in the conclusion chapter). However, in giving conference presentations on various aspects of the research, the researchers summarised what they did in a slide entitled 'Research Questions', with a set of questions that were retrospectively fitted to the analyses that were carried out. So, for example, a presentation which focussed on stigmatising and change over time contained an early slide with the following questions:

1. How do different newspapers represent people with obesity?
2. What legitimation strategies are used with negative representations?

3. Has stigmatising language decreased over time?
4. In what other ways has discourse around obesity changed over time?

There is considerable freedom in naming the research questions at the end of a project, along with allowing them to develop organically through a combination of reading around the topic, conversations with others, exploratory corpus procedures, or simply following hunches or analytical paths that look potentially interesting. However, as we will see in the rest of this chapter, there are other ways to develop research questions, which may bring with them unforeseen advantages.

2.3 Developing Questions in Interaction with Stakeholders

In this section we turn to a project where interactions with healthcare practitioners led to the formulation of research questions that could be answered by means of corpus linguistic methods. In this case the focus was a language-based questionnaire for the diagnosis of pain: the McGill Pain Questionnaire (MPQ; Melzack, 1975). To contextualise this project, we start by providing some background on pain, the diagnosis of pain, and the role of language within it. We then introduce the MPQ and the issues associated with it that led to the formulation of research questions which were suitable for a corpus linguistic approach, as part of a collaboration between linguists and a pain clinician (Semino et al., 2020).

Pain can have a wide variety of causes. A fundamental distinction can, however, be made between *nociceptive* and *neuropathic* pain. Nociceptive pain is caused by damage to bodily tissues, as in the case of cuts, burns, and fractures (Vadivelu et al., 2011). As such, nociceptive pain is arguably the most 'prototypical' kind of pain. Other things being equal, it is also relatively straightforward to diagnose, as it is possible to identify its cause by observation through the naked eye or medical tests such as X-rays or scans. In contrast, neuropathic pain is not, or not only, the result of bodily damage but is caused by problems in the nervous system that may not be easily observable, including via X-rays or scans (Wilkie et al., 2001). Neuropathic pain also tends to become chronic (i.e., to last more than three months). The most extreme example of neuropathic pain is phantom limb pain, which is experienced in a limb that the person no longer has (e.g., following amputation). But more common types of pain, such as headaches and back pain, can have a neuropathic component and thus be difficult to diagnose and treat. The *way* in which the patient describes their pain– what it feels like (its 'quality') and how bad it is (its 'severity' or 'intensity') – is always important in healthcare settings, but it is particularly crucial in the case of neuropathic pain, especially when it is chronic.

2.3 Developing Questions in Interaction with Stakeholders   21

Expressing pain in language is, however, notoriously difficult (e.g., Scarry, 1987). In English, for example, the set of lexical items that have literal meanings relating to pain is relatively small and non-specific (e.g., *pain/painful*, *hurt* as noun and verb, *sore*, and *ache/aching*). Consequently, pain is often expressed figuratively. Neuropathic pain particularly tends to be expressed metaphorically in terms of causes of damage to the body (Semino, 2010). For example, we talk about a 'burning pain' in the stomach when there is no fire or a 'splitting headache' when our head is not split.

Against this background, clinicians have developed language-based tools for the diagnosis of pain, such as the MPQ, which is reproduced in Figure 2.1. The MPQ was developed at McGill University in Canada in the 1970s. As the figure shows, it includes 78 possible English linguistic descriptors of pain divided into 20 groups, each consisting of between 2 and 7 descriptors. The division into groups is central to the goal of the questionnaire, which was to capture both the *quality* and *severity* of the patient's pain (i.e., what the pain feels like and how intense it is). The groups capture different qualities or types of pain and fall into four broader classes, depending on the aspect of pain they reflect: sensory (groups 1–10), affective (groups 11–15), evaluative (group 16), and miscellaneous (groups 17–20). Within each group, the descriptors are listed in order of increasing severity or intensity of pain. For example, group 3 captures the sensory quality of *punctate pressure* and contains five descriptors: *pricking*, *boring*, *drilling*, *stabbing*, and *lancinating*. *Pricking* is the descriptor associated with the lowest severity within the group, and *lancinating* is associated with the highest intensity. Group 3 is also one of several groups of descriptors that consist of metaphorical descriptions of the quality of pain in terms of different causes of damage to the body.

When completing the questionnaire, patients have two options with regard to each group: they may not pick any of the descriptors, if that quality of pain does not apply to them (e.g., if their pain does not feel hot, they do not pick any descriptors from group 7); alternatively, if the relevant quality of pain does apply to them, they pick *one* descriptor (namely, according to the design of the questionnaire, the one that best captures the severity of that kind of pain). In this way, by looking at a patient's selections, the clinician has an overview of both the kind(s) of pain that the patient experiences and their intensity.

A few years prior to the writing of this book, one of the authors (ES), who has an interest in communication about pain, was asked for advice about the MPQ by a pain clinician (Dr Joanna Zakzrewska) who regularly employs the questionnaire in her consultations with patients, alongside other approaches aimed at diagnosing the cause of their pain. The clinician reported that her patients sometimes struggled with some of the descriptors included in the MPQ and/or found it difficult to select a single descriptor from the groups that applied to their experience of pain. Indeed, to avoid multiple selections from each group,

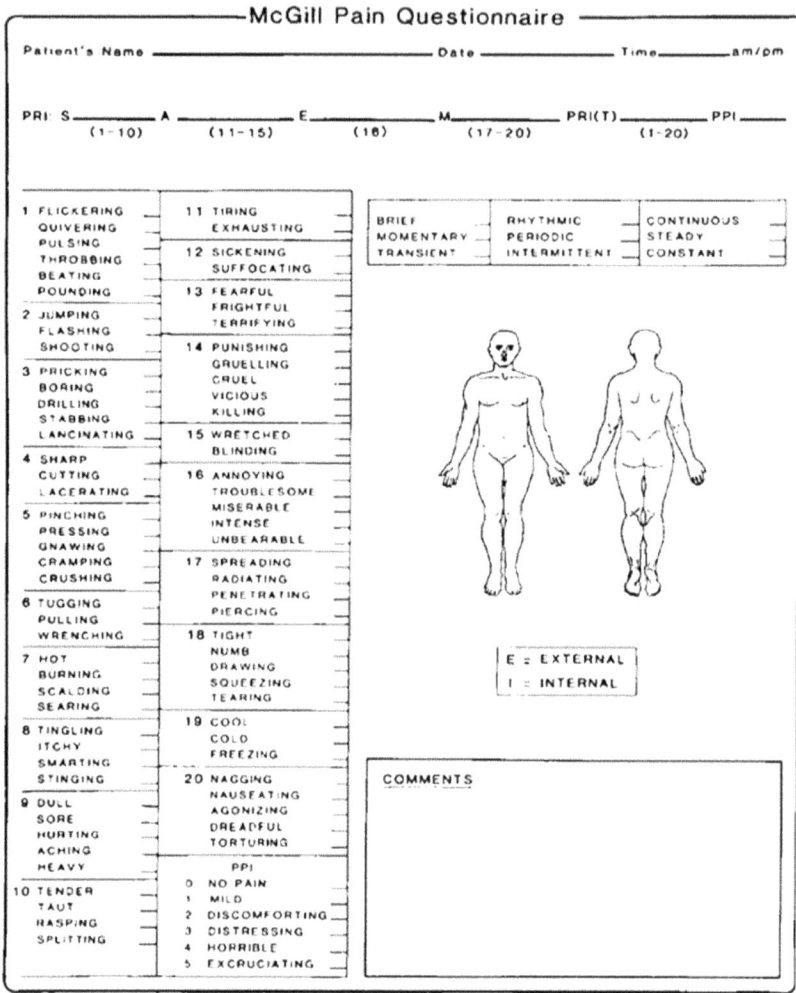

Figure 2.1 The McGill Pain Questionnaire. (MPQ; Melzack, 1983: 44)

this clinician administered the MPQ verbally (i.e., reading out each group to the patient and asking them to select one descriptor only per group). The clinician therefore wondered whether a linguistic perspective on the MPQ might explain the problems encountered by her patients.

As we have explained, the MPQ relies on two dimensions of variation between the 78 descriptors: across groups, there is intended to be variation in terms of pain

2.3 Developing Questions in Interaction with Stakeholders

quality; within each group, there is intended to be variation in terms of pain severity. Even before carrying out any analysis, a linguist might expect that the 78 descriptors are likely to contrast in other ways. However, before attempting to turn the clinician's general question into a set of viable research questions for a corpus linguist, previous studies on the MPQ itself needed to be considered.

The MPQ has been widely used in pain diagnosis, both in its original English language version and in translations into at least 26 additional languages. On one hand, its application to a wide range of conditions has shown that it is a valid, reliable, and sensitive tool. According to a systematic review by Main (2016: 1390), 'there is evidence that the MPQ (1) can discriminate between pain conditions, and also capture variation within conditions, (2) is sensitive to change, and (3) is responsive to treatment and can be used as an outcome measure'. On the other hand, a number of studies have pointed out issues with the MPQ descriptors, including that some are rare words in English (e.g., *rasping*), some may be ambiguous (e.g., *boring*, from the *punctate pressure* group above), and some may not often be used to describe pain (e.g., *taut*; Fernandez and Boyle, 2002). Partly as a result of these issues, two shorter versions of the MPQ have been produced since the launch of the original one: Short-Form-MPQ (SF-MPQ; Melzack, 1987) and Short-Form-MPQ-2 (SF-MPQ-2; Dworkin et al., 2009). The first, SF-MPQ, was developed as a less-time-consuming version of the original MPQ and contains 15 descriptors, each rated on a 4-point intensity scale. The second, SF-MPQ-2, contains 7 additional items intended to be relevant to neuropathic pain (i.e., pain caused by problems in the nervous system) and adopts a 10-point scale for pain intensity.

Against this background, it was then possible to identify two main dimensions of variation among the 78 descriptors that would be possible to investigate by means of corpus methods to address the clinician's concern, and to contribute a new linguistic perspective to existing literature:

- the frequency of each descriptor in English, which can be taken as a proxy measure of each word's familiarity for patients;
- the tendency for each descriptor to be used to describe pain, which can be operationalised in terms of the corpus linguistic notion of collocation.

This led to the formulation of the following research questions:

1. To what extent do the 78 descriptors included in the McGill Pain Questionnaire vary in terms of their frequency in general English?
2. To what extent do the 78 descriptors included in the McGill Pain Questionnaire vary in terms of the strength of collocation with the string *pain*?

Answering these questions required the selection of a suitable corpus of English. The Oxford English Corpus (OEC) was selected for this purpose. The OEC includes 2.5 billion words of twenty-first-century English. It is mainly drawn from material collected from the World Wide Web and contains texts from a wide range of genres and domains (e.g., news and media, law, medicine, science, business, fiction, personal blogs). It also includes texts from international varieties of English from different parts of the world (e.g., UK, US, Australia, India, Singapore). As such, it is an appropriate reference corpus of 'general English'. The OEC is accessible and searchable via the corpus manager and text analysis software Sketch Engine (www.sketchengine.eu; Kilgarriff et al., 2014).

Semino and colleagues (2020) show how answering question 1 above revealed substantial variation in the frequency of the MPQ descriptors in the OEC. The most frequent MPQ descriptor, *hot*, occurs 206,291 times in the OEC (84.857 instances per million words), while the least frequent, *lancinating*, occurs only 15 times (0.006 instances per million words) and only appears in medical research articles about the MPQ itself. More generally, answering question 2 identifies a set of 15 MPQ descriptors that occur less than once per million words in the OEC (e.g., *quivering, smarting*, and *taut*) and thus can be considered relatively rare words. This provided the pain clinician with evidence of what words her patients are more likely to find difficult to understand.

Semino and colleagues (2020) also found considerable variation in the strength of collocation between each descriptor and the word *pain* in the OEC. As part of this, they showed, for example, that *sharp* has 986 co-occurrences with the lemma *pain* as a noun (in a window of 5 words to the left and 5 words to the right of the descriptor), while *rasping* has none. More broadly, 24 descriptors were found to have 10 or fewer instances of *pain* within the relevant collocational window in the whole corpus, including *flashing, jumping, sickening*, and *tugging*. Collocation is a linguistic phenomenon, but it has been hypothesised to reflect psychological associations between words in our mental lexicons (Hoey, 2005), which can lead to 'priming effects', whereby being exposed to one member of a collocational pair leads to faster recognition of the other member of the pair in experimental settings. In the MPQ, however, any such priming effects could be problematic, as the patient's selections within each group of descriptors are taken to reflect the severity of the patient's pain. This led to the formulation of a third research question:

3. To what extent does variation in the strength of collocation with 'pain' within each of the 20 groups in the McGill Pain Questionnaire correlate with patients' selections for each group?

To answer this question, Semino and colleagues (2020) brought together two sources of data: patients' selections in 800 completed questionnaires at the Eastman Dental Hospital in London and information about the strength of collocation between each descriptor and the noun lemma *pain* in the OEC. Using a standard measure of correlation (the Pearson correlation coefficient), they found that for 7 out of 10 sensory groups in the MPQ, patients' choice of descriptor can be explained largely or entirely in terms of the strength of the collocational link from the word *pain* to that descriptor. For example, in group 2, patients overwhelmingly selected *shooting*, which has a much stronger collocational link with *pain* than the other descriptors and, within the MPQ, is at the top of the severity scale. In group 4, patients overwhelmingly selected *sharp*, which also has a much stronger collocational link with *pain* than the other descriptors but, within the MPQ, is at the bottom of the severity scale.

This finding undermines the reliability of the original version of the MPQ for the measurement of pain severity and goes some way towards explaining why, in the experience of the pain clinician mentioned at the beginning of this section, patients may find it difficult to pick just one descriptor from at least some of the groups. As the two short-form MPQs approach pain severity differently (via a numerical score associated with each descriptor), the answer to research question 3 also suggests that these versions of the questionnaires may be more appropriate for that purpose.

In summary, this section has shown how a language-related problem in healthcare can lead to the formulation of research questions suitable for corpus linguistic methods, and how answering these questions can help address the original problem. The process of developing research questions is fairly typical of corpus-based studies of health communication that develop from interactions between healthcare professionals/researchers and linguists. A possible disadvantage of this approach is that the resulting research questions are not driven by the interests or priorities of linguists, and thus they may not lead to major new insights into language or discourse. On the other hand, as we have shown, answering research questions formulated in interaction with stakeholders can result in findings that have immediate practical relevance. In addition, the process of answering such questions can sometimes require some useful adaptation or development of corpus methods themselves. For example, Semino and colleagues (2020) used a two-pronged approach to collocation in the MPQ study. In Chapter 10 we discuss a study of the representation of hallucinatory voices that required the development of an ad hoc corpus linguistic approach to the analysis of social actors in interview data.

The next section further explores the potential advantages and disadvantages of addressing questions raised by practitioners, by presenting a study where the analytical focus is far more strictly governed from the outset.

2.4 Working with a Set of Pregiven Questions from Non-academic Partners

In this section we outline a study (described in more detail in Baker et al., 2019) where the analysts had limited freedom when it came to decisions about the focus of the project and the subsequent direction of the analysis. When working with external agents, it is often the case that the researcher will be required to address a set of predetermined goals, which may be non-negotiable requirements in exchange for access to a particular corpus. There are potential benefits and pitfalls to this kind of relationship: embarking on a piece of new research with a ready-made dataset and a clear set of preset goals could save time, and there is less need to engage with exploratory forms of research in order to identify areas of interest. However, the questions set by people who have not used corpus linguistics methods before might also be difficult to answer, as we began to show in the previous section. They may not be worded in ways that enable research to be carried out appropriately or effectively; in addition, the kinds of questions being asked might overlook other important aspects of the data.

In 2015, members of the Centre for Corpus Approaches to Social Science (CASS) were contacted by a senior member of the Patients and Information Directorate at NHS England. This section of the NHS was involved with analysing patient feedback which had been posted to a website. At the time, a set of almost 29 million words in comments from patients, along with 11.6 million words in responses from NHS providers, was publicly available, consisting of posts made between March 2013 and September 2015. The researchers at CASS were asked if they would consider carrying out a corpus-assisted discourse analysis of these posts, in order to help NHS England make sense of such a large amount of data, as well as to develop methods of analysis which could be shared with staff at NHS England, so that they could analyse large amounts of feedback in the future. A proviso was that NHS England would provide a set of questions, and the team at CASS would be required to produce detailed reports within 18 months to answer these questions.

The researchers were duly presented with 12 questions which had been compiled during a team meeting at the Patients and Information Directorate (CASS members were not present at this meeting). The team admitted that not all of their members had seen the corpus data in advance, so some of them had struggled a little to devise questions. They conveyed that they were also happy for the members of CASS to consider any additional aspects of interest that emerged as they carried out their analysis. The questions that were set by the NHS team are listed as follows:

1. What are the key drivers for positive and negative feedback?
2. What are the key differences in experience across different providers (e.g., acute providers and General Practitioners)?
3. How consistent are the messages within a provider (or site, department ward, if available)?
4. Are the comments consistent with the quantitative ratings/scores?

2.4 Pregiven Questions from Non-academic Partners

5. What are the main areas of concern / what matters most to patients (e.g., relational or functional aspects of care)?
6. Who is the focus of the concern raised (e.g., individual staff member – nurse, General Practitioners, general/organisational)?
7. What impact has the experience had on the individual posting a comment?
8. What is the 'quality' of the comments provided (e.g., content, length, clarity, relevance, specificity)?
9. Are there any differences by socio-demographic group?
10. What key words within a text might trigger an alert/urgent review?
11. Can the comments be easily categorised (e.g., positive/negative, important/urgent)?
12. What proportion of comments say something along the lines of 'I've already raised this and you've done nothing about it' (i.e., repeat/ongoing concerns)?

Some of the questions are worded in ways that would suggest a yes/no answer (e.g., questions 4, 9, and 11), something which the researchers on this project would tend to avoid in their own research, instead preferring a wording which allows for a more open answer. For example, question 4 could be rephrased as 'to what extent, and how are the comments consistent with quantitative ratings/scores?' Several questions contained comparative aspects (e.g., questions 1, 2, 4, and 9), which are generally well-suited to corpus-assisted techniques of analysis. Some questions referred to more vague criteria, such as question 3, which referred to 'messages'; question 7, which referred to the impact on the individual; question 10, which referred to words that might trigger an urgent review; and question 12, which referred to repeated or ongoing concerns. A potential disadvantage of corpus-based approaches is that it can be difficult to search and retrieve all cases of a variable linguistic item. For example, there are many ways that someone can indicate that they have raised a concern before. And sometimes simply searching for what appears to be the most obvious phrasings will produce little value. For example, the phrases 'I have raised this concern before' and 'I have already raised this' did not occur at all in the patient feedback corpus. In particular, question 10 raised another question: what kind of problems in the NHS would require an alert or urgent review, and would the criteria for this be qualitative (e.g., something terrible happening), quantitative (e.g., something happening often), or both?

When the researchers at CASS received the list of questions, they found some of them to be more challenging than others, and they reasoned that most of these questions would probably not have been ones that they would have asked of the data, when relying on corpus methods. However, perhaps this could be seen as a positive aspect of working with external partners. The partners did not have a sense of what was easy (or not) for a corpus-assisted discourse analysis, so their questions were based on what they felt was important to know, rather than being restricted by considerations regarding what they thought the tools could tell us. And these 'difficult' questions were interesting in that they required the corpus researchers to work outside their comfort zone, to think creatively about the possible ways that they could be addressed.

The CASS researchers read samples of the corpus in order to identify cases where language was used in relation to the more variable phenomena. For example, question 7 asked about the impact of an experience on a patient, and after some experimentation, it was decided to consider impact in terms of the feelings that the patient described, along with expressions of their intentions. This led to the consideration of phrases like 'I will/will not/won't' and 'I feel'. It was found that the former set of phrases collocated with verbs like *change*, *move*, *leave*, *return*, *recommend*, and *forget*. Examination of concordance lines containing these kinds of collocates helped identify the kinds of cases where patients said they were intending to change their provider and under what circumstances (e.g., poor standard of treatment, long wait times, poor staff interpersonal skills, lack of medication availability) and cases where patients said that they would (or not) recommend the provider to others. Examination of collocates of 'I feel' uncovered examples of people describing how they felt 'let down', 'sorry', 'fortunate', or 'safe', and subsequent concordance analyses were able to provide further detail regarding the reasons for these feelings. There are undoubtedly other ways that patients can talk about their intentions and feelings, but the researchers had identified a set of seed phrases that produced reasonably large enough cases for them to be able to conduct an analysis. The solution, then, was not to identify every phrasing but to find frequently used phrasings that were employed by a range of different people and could be taken as reasonably representative.

What the CASS team found interesting about engaging with the NHS feedback was that a relatively simple research question about demographic differences led to the formulation of a related and more complex set of research questions, regarding what happens when people reveal information about their age or gender, and whether such cases are representative of the kinds of concerns their peer group generally has. These other questions could not be answered using just the original corpus, but the experiences of the initial study could be used to inform a later set of research questions for a follow-up study.

Indeed, one aspect of trying to answer the research questions that had been set by the NHS team was that the researchers realised that they were also answering a set of questions that they had not initially thought of and also had not been suggested by the NHS. A clue to these kinds of questions can be found if we look to feedback provided by two female patients, aged 20 and 83 years. In these cases, it was found that the patients were using aspects of their identity as a way of

2.4 Pregiven Questions from Non-academic Partners

justifying or legitimating their position. As the analyses pertaining to the original 12 research questions were carried out, more cases were found where patients used language in various ways in order to represent themselves as worthy of attention or simply as being in the right. Three examples of these incidents are as follows:

> The nurse who saw me they were the rudest person I've ever come across in my life, they came out and shouted to the reception why I was I given the appointment as I was late they were shouting so I could hear, and when they called me in, they made me apologise I'm a married man with two kids.

> Been going there 12 yrs & rarely darken their doors. I am now left with what seems like placebo medication and disinclined to go back.

> My family also have been with [anonymised] Surgery ever since one was introduced, we have been a long standing and well respected family in the parish for over 400 years but, obviously this counts for nothing these days!

In the first example, the patient criticises a nurse who shouted to reception about him being late for his appointment, and then notes that he was made to apologise. At the end of his criticism, he provides his marital status and notes that he has two children. He doesn't elaborate on why this statement is relevant. A possible interpretation of the patient's self-description is that these aspects of his identity indicate that he is a 'grown-up' and thus he was unfairly treated like a child when made to apologise. Additionally, the statement might be interpreted as the patient implying that he should not be blamed for being late due to the responsibilities that come with fatherhood. In the second case, the patient constructs themself as a 'good patient' as opposed to someone who continually seeks medical help by mentioning that they 'rarely darken their doors'. Thus, they construct themself as someone who is able to give a credible opinion. Finally, the patient in the third example notes that they are from a family which has been respected locally for more than 400 years, a point which they relate with disappointment that it 'counts for nothing'.

It was found that patients regularly participated in this kind of legitimation work, and that there was evidence that different legitimation strategies were employed by different demographic groups. This aspect of the feedback was highlighted to the NHS, as it was reasoned that it is important to have awareness of these kinds of strategies, and to ensure that some forms of feedback are not privileged at the expense of others, just because some people are better at using certain strategies to strengthen the impact of their messages. Awareness about the potential power of legitimation strategies can therefore be important, as service providers need to make decisions about which kinds of feedback to respond to and in what ways.

The example relating to legitimation strategies was just one way that the researchers discovered they were answering questions that they had not originally planned to address. As a result, after answering the 12 questions put forward by NHS England, the researchers added 4 new questions to the original list (see Baker et al., 2019):

13. Why do patients leave feedback?
14. What does the language of patients reveal about their expectations?
15. How do patients use language to construct their positions as legitimate?
16. What discourses do service providers draw on when responding to patient feedback?

A final aspect to mention about this study relates to timing. As previously noted, this project lasted 18 months and the researchers were given 12 questions to address. This is somewhat different from other corpus-assisted discourse analysis projects, where researchers are generally able to set their own questions or even to start the work with no questions. It was calculated that, taking holidays and weekends into account, the researchers would have about 28 working days to address each question by devising methods to analyse the data, then conducting the analysis and writing up the results. This was not a lot of time, and while they were able to provide reports for each question, it was felt that for some questions, more time would have been preferable in order to provide a more accurate or detailed set of responses. The NHS contacts were happy with the results that were given to them (so much so that they asked members of CASS to look at a second set of feedback, discussed in Chapter 10), and they did not make unreasonable demands relating to deadlines.

However, with other external partners there were perhaps somewhat unrealistic expectations regarding what members of CASS could produce within short timeframes (including expectations that they would work weekends in order to provide reports for meetings on Monday mornings). A key aspect of working with external partners, then, is to provide clear expectations about the amount of work that researchers are able to carry out within a given timeframe and the kinds of questions that can be answered easily (or not). A good organisation will be happy to view this kind of research as collaborative and as consisting of a dialogue where expectations on both sides may need to be adjusted occasionally. With that said, there was a definite benefit to having questions and deadlines set in advance by external partners, one which was perhaps not obvious from the outset but which became clearer as the project progressed.

2.5 Conclusion

Research questions are a central part of the process of doing research. As we have shown, however, different projects may involve different approaches to the development of research questions, with researchers potentially becoming involved at different points and being able to exercise different amounts of

2.5 Conclusion

control on the nature of the questions. This applies particularly when doing research that crosses boundaries between disciplines and/or that involves interactions between researchers and practitioners, as in the case of our research on health communication. In addition, the power and flexibility of corpus linguistic methods make them potentially suitable and attractive for a wide variety of questions, data, and stakeholders, resulting in the different kinds of experiences we have presented.

Other things being equal, researchers may always wish for the freedom of exploration that we have described in relation to the study on media representation of obesity. However, we hope to have shown the value of considering the challenges and compromises involved in answering questions formulated more or less strictly by, in our case, people working in healthcare. Both the second and third case study resulted in findings relevant to practice and/or policy, they helped strengthen the relationships between CASS and valuable partners, and they forced CASS researchers to adapt and stretch their corpus linguistic expertise in ways that were interesting and more beneficial beyond each specific project.

The rest of this book will continue to show how doing corpus research on health communication often tested our ability to be flexible, adaptable, and creative not just at the start of the process but throughout. We will also continue to show how rewarding these experiences have been. In the next chapter, we turn to the topic of collecting data for the purposes of corpus construction.

References

Baker, P. and Brookes, G. (2022). *Analysing Language, Sex and Age in a Corpus of Patient Feedback: A Comparison of Approaches*. Cambridge University Press.

Baker, P., Brookes, G. and Evans, C. (2019). *The Language of Patient Feedback: A Corpus Linguistic Study of Online Health Communication*. Routledge.

Baker, P., Gabrielatos, C. and McEnery, T. (2013). *Discourse Analysis and Media Attitudes: The Representation of Islam in the British Press*. Cambridge University Press.

Bettini, M. (1995). *I classici nell'età dell'indiscrezione*. Einaudi.

Bordo, S. R. (1993). *Unbearable Weight: Feminism, Western Culture, and the Body*. University of California Press.

Brookes, G. and Baker, P. (2021). *Obesity in the News: Language and Representation in the Press*. Cambridge University Press.

Dworkin, R. H., Turk, D. C., Revicki, D. A., Harding, G., Coyne, K. S., Peirce-Sander, S., Bhagwat, D., Everton, D., Burke, L. B., Cowan, P., Farrar, J. T., Hertz, S., Max, M. B., Rappaport, B. A. and Melzack, R. (2009). Development and Initial Validation of an Expanded and Revised Version of the Short-Form McGill Pain Questionnaire (SF-MPQ-2). *Pain*, *144*, 35–42. https://doi.org/10.1016/j.pain.2009.02.007.

Fernandez, E. and Boyle, G. J. (2002). Affective and Evaluative Descriptors of Pain in the McGill Pain Questionnaire: Reduction and Reorganization. *Journal of Pain*, *3* (1), 70–7. https://doi.org/10.1054/jpai.2001.xbcorr25530.

Gill, R., Henwood, K. and McLean, C. (2000). The Tyranny of the 'Six-Pack'? Culture in Psychology. In C. Squire (ed.), *Culture in Psychology* (pp. 100–17). Routledge.

Glaser, B. G. and Strauss, A. (1967). *The Discovery of Grounded Theory: Strategies for Qualitative Research*. Aldine.

Gough, B. (2010). Promoting 'Masculinity' over Health: A Critical Analysis of Men's Health Promotion with Particular Reference to an Obesity Reduction Manual. In B. Gough and S. Robertson (eds.), *Men, Masculinities and Health: Critical Perspectives* (pp. 125–42). Palgrave Macmillan.

Gries, S. Th. (2011). Quantitative and Exploratory Corpus Approaches to Registers and Text Types. Plenary given at Corpus Linguistics 2011, University of Birmingham, 20–2, July 2011.

Hoey, M. (2005). *Lexical Priming: A New Theory of Words and Language*. Routledge.

Kilgarriff, A., Baisa, V., Bušta, J., Jakubíček, M., Kovář, V., Michelfeit, J., Rychlý, P. and Suchomel, V. (2014). The Sketch Engine: Ten Years On. *Lexicography*, *1*, 7–36. https://doi.org/10.1007/s40607-014-0009-9.

Main, C. J. (2016). Pain Assessment in Context: A State of the Science Review of the McGill Pain Questionnaire 40 Years On. *Pain*, 157(7): 1387–99.

Marchi, A. (2014). A Corpus-Assisted Study of the Guardian's View on Journalism. Unpublished PhD thesis. Lancaster University.

Melzack R. (1975). The McGill Pain Questionnaire: Major Properties and Scoring Methods. *Pain*, *1*, 277–99. https://doi.org/10.1016/0304-3959(75)90044-5.

(1983). The McGill Pain Questionnaire. In R. Melzack (ed.), *Pain Measurement and Assessment* (pp. 41–7). Raven Press.

(1987). The Short-Form McGill Pain Questionnaire. *Pain*, *30*, 191–7. https://doi.org/10.1016/0304-3959(87)91074-8.

Scarry, E. (1987). *The Body in Pain: The Making and Unmaking of the World*. Oxford University Press.

Semino, E. (2010). Descriptions of Pain, Metaphor and Embodied Simulation. *Metaphor and Symbol*, *25*(4), 205–26. https://doi.org/10.1080/10926488.2010.510926.

Semino, E., Hardie, A. and Zakzrwska, J. M. (2020). Applying Corpus Linguistics to a Diagnostic Tool for Pain. In Z. Demjén (ed.), *Applying Linguistics in Illness and Healthcare Contexts* (pp. 99–128). Bloomsbury.

Sunderland, J. (2010). Research Questions in Linguistics. In L. Litosseliti (ed.), *Research Methods in Linguistics* (pp. 9–28). Continuum.

Vadivelu, N., Urman, R. D. and Hines, R. L. (2011). *Essentials of Pain Management*. Springer.

Wilkie, D. G., Huan, H.-Y., Reilly, N. and Cain, K. C. (2001). Nociceptive and Neuropathic Pain in Patients with Lung Cancer: A Comparison of Pain Quality Descriptors. *Journal of Pain and Symptom Management*, *22*(5), 899–910. https://doi.org/10.1016/s0885-3924(01)00351-7.

Wray, A. and Bloomer, A. (2021). *Projects in Linguistics and Language Studies*, 3rd ed. Routledge.

3 Collecting Data

3.1 Introduction

In this chapter we reflect on different approaches to identifying the data that we analyse using corpus methods, since data selection has significant implications for the kinds of observations that we can make about health communication. (For a general introduction to corpus construction, see Reppen (2022).) As a fundamental part of the research process, it pays to approach data collection early on. That being said, our research aims, what we know from our reading of the relevant literature and what types of health communication are available for study can all inform how we identify, collect and record data. We report on three different approaches to data collection that utilise language content that is variously 'ready-made' for corpus analysis; in doing so, we demonstrate how the construction of corpora is often guided by research imperatives, practical and ethical concerns (see also Chapter 4), and data formatting.

The aspects of data collection discussed in this chapter will be pertinent to any kind of corpus construction, though there are particular concerns relating to the highly sensitive and personal nature of health communication data. We must also consider the extent to which the presence of a researcher in naturally occurring health communication contexts might disrupt and therefore have unfavourable impacts on the delivery of healthcare. Nevertheless, documenting healthcare interactions in their most naturally occurring state, along with relevant contextual metadata, is crucial for generating insights that can contribute to the optimisation of care.

Although we can refer to large, general corpora to investigate how, for example, people discuss health topics in general conversation, the corpora used in health-related research are most likely to be specialised. It is often the case that such corpora are purpose-built for the study, requiring some thought in terms of their design and construction. Targeting specific kinds of health content can mitigate the extent to which the corpus is representative of the perspectives of a general population. On the other hand, the population might also be targeted for its specialisation; for instance, we might want to focus on the contributions of those who have lived experience of the health topic.

Specialisation may also refer to a specific time period, though with historical data, we may be further restricted simply to what is available – a concern that is not exclusive to health topics.

The case studies discussed in this chapter focus on the preparation of data for the purposes of corpus-assisted research. In other words, they reflect the efforts of the researchers in facilitating analytical procedures germane to corpus analysis. To this end, we consider questions relating to what texts should be included in the corpus, how much data is required and how the files in the corpus should be organised. We reflect on the impacts of preparing those files in a machine-readable format, accounting for our decision-making on what features of the texts to include and whether we apply any kind of annotation. Finally, we discuss the importance of associated metadata and how this is incorporated into the corpus design, to enrich our interpretation of the corpus outputs.

In reporting our different approaches to data collection and corpus construction, we set out to inform readers of the key moments when it is beneficial to reflect on the purposes of the research and offer a view of some of the options that can help make this process more efficient and productive for those research purposes. We begin by looking at the fundamentals of creating a new dataset to investigate representations of obesity.

3.2 Compiling a News Corpus about Obesity

The first corpus we discuss in this chapter is the one constructed by Brookes and Baker (2021) for their analysis of how obesity is discursively represented in UK newspapers. In particular, we describe the processes and critical considerations that were involved in designing and constructing this relatively large (approximately 36 million words), purpose-built corpus of health-related media language.

3.2.1 Selecting Texts: Representativeness and Balance

When designing a corpus, one of our first considerations is what kinds of texts and language use we want it to represent. This decision, like all considerations underpinning corpus design, will be driven first and foremost by our research questions and/or the broader purpose of our corpus. However, in most cases, we as researchers and corpus builders do not have access to – or even complete knowledge of – the full extent of the texts that could be deemed relevant for our research purposes, even if these purposes are very clearly defined.[1] For this reason, most corpora constitute a mere sample of all the possible texts 'out

---

[1] Exceptions to this are corpora that are designed to represent so-called closed text types, where all the possible texts are known to us (e.g., if we were studying the published works of a deceased author).

3.2 Compiling a News Corpus about Obesity

there' that could have been included. We will therefore typically have to decide how we are going to sample texts from all the possible language use 'out there' in the world that could suit our purposes and help us answer our research questions. Designing a corpus essentially involves developing a sampling frame to help us decide which texts will be included in the corpus and whether we will include these texts in their entirety or sample material from them (Biber, 2004: 174).

At this point, considerations around representativeness become relevant. Biber (1993: 244) defines representativeness as 'the extent to which a sample includes the full range of variability in a population'. Here the term 'population' refers not necessarily to a group of people but more conceptually to the 'notional space within which language is being sampled' (McEnery and Hardie, 2012: 8). Broadly speaking, the more representative of the target population our sample (or corpus) is, the greater confidence we can have that our findings can be generalised to the population under study.

In assembling a corpus of news reporting about obesity, Brookes and Baker (2021) had to decide what they wanted their data to represent and then design their corpus accordingly. They wanted to assemble British articles that covered the topic of obesity, so they searched for articles using the LexisNexis online news archive, which stores digitised versions of online and print editions of newspaper articles from a range of countries, including the UK. Brookes and Baker (2021) searched for all articles containing one or more mentions of the word *obese* and/or *obesity*. This is a relatively liberal search criterion, compared to corpus studies of news texts more broadly (which often stipulate that search terms need to occur multiple times and/or within the headline or lead paragraph; e.g., Brookes, 2023). Brookes and Baker's more liberal search criteria had the advantage that it yielded a larger number of results. A potential disadvantage of this approach is that it yields a considerable number of articles that are not 'about' obesity but which, rather, mention it in passing. (For a discussion of 'aboutness', see Scott and Tribble (2006); for ways of measuring aboutness in the process of corpus design, see Scott (2017).) Yet, viewed another way, their decision to include such cases brought the analytical advantage that it allowed the researchers to consider instances in which obesity was, in being mentioned in passing, accordingly 'topicalised' within the context of reporting around other news topics and events. It could also be argued that every mention of a topic, even briefly, will contribute towards the incremental effect of discourse around that topic.

As noted, Brookes and Baker (2021) decided to focus on contemporary UK coverage on obesity, and they defined 'contemporary' as the last 10 years prior to the start of their research. For this reason, they searched for articles published between 2008 and 2017 (inclusive). Had they wanted to adopt a more historical focus, they would have had to sample texts from further into the past. This would also have influenced how they went about sourcing texts for the corpus; while LexisNexis provides reliable coverage of recent years, this coverage becomes patchier as we go further back in time – meaning that this repository is not ideally suited for researching historical news texts.

Even once the researchers had decided that they wanted to focus on UK coverage, and within that to adopt a contemporary focus, the British press still holds a lot of variation that the authors needed to consider when building the corpus. Newspapers in the UK can be distinguished according to their coverage (i.e., national, regional), their format or 'style' (i.e., broadsheet, tabloid), their political stance (i.e., left-leaning, right-leaning or centrist) and their frequency of appearance (i.e., daily, weekly).

Brookes and Baker (2021) decided to focus on national as opposed to regional coverage (due to time limits on how much they could analyse). They included both broadsheets and tabloids, and newspapers across the political spectrum. In terms of frequency, they focused on daily newspapers but included as part of this each newspaper's Sunday, online and so-called sister editions. For example, when collecting texts from the *Daily Mail*, they included texts from the *Mail Online* and *Mail on Sunday*. This marked an important way in which Brookes and Baker sought to expand on previous research on the topic, which had focussed, in the main (and in the context of the UK, exclusively), on printed newspapers only. Table 3.1 gives a breakdown of the article and word counts for each newspaper in the corpus, as well as the mean article length for each newspaper.

As this table shows, Brookes and Baker's corpus was not equally balanced in terms of the number of articles and words contributed by each newspaper. One newspaper, the *Mail*, contributed around 30 per cent of the words in the

Table 3.1 *Number of articles, words, and mean article lengths in Brookes and Baker's (2021) corpus*

Newspaper	Articles	Words	Mean article length (in words)
Express	5,193	3,265,741	629
Guardian	5,008	5,238,062	1,046
Independent	4,336	3,303,269	762
Mail	12,805	11,890,340	929
Mirror	3,398	2,202,323	648
Morning Star	152	63,641	419
Star	1,072	370,818	346
Sun	2,286	1,082,808	474
Telegraph	5,680	4,804,351	846
Times	3,948	3,831,868	971
Total	**43,878**	**36,053,221**	**822**

3.2 Compiling a News Corpus about Obesity

corpus, while the contribution of the *Morning Star* is marginal. Average article length also varied considerably, with the *Guardian*'s average being more than double that of tabloids such as the *Star* and *Sun*. Such imbalances are important to acknowledge, and researchers can make adaptations to their sampling frame to regularise the contributions coming from different sources. (See Baker (2009) for a discussion of the design of the Brown family of reference corpora.) Rather than take, for example, 500-word samples from articles, Brookes and Baker (2021) decided to include all texts in their entirety, on the basis that the functions of the representational discourses they identified could be generated across the full length of the text(s) in question. With respect to the imbalance in the number of articles from each newspaper, they argued that this represented the real-life press landscape and, more specifically, the corresponding imbalance in terms of how much obesity coverage is provided by each of the newspapers they sampled. This imbalance did not pose much of an issue for their analysis, since Brookes and Baker (2021) compared different newspapers and sections of the press using relative rather than raw frequency information. Nevertheless, it is important to acknowledge that in such cases, what can be determined from the corpus is based on the language used in some newspapers that are represented more than others. Accordingly, they modulated any claims based on their analysis of the whole corpus with this imbalance in mind.

Once the relevant texts have been identified, researchers can structure their corpus in such a way as to facilitate queries and comparisons at various levels. Brookes and Baker (2021) downloaded and stored the articles in their corpus in a way that would allow them to discriminate at the level of the text. This allowed them to carry out comparisons of the articles according to their format (i.e., broadsheets versus tabloids), political leaning (i.e., left-leaning versus right-leaning), and date of publication (i.e., looking at change over time). In addition to having analytical utility, this method of storing data also allowed Brookes and Baker to assess the balance and representativeness of their corpus (and, in turn, to modulate their analytical claims), in a way that would not have been possible (or at least practical) had they stored their corpus data in a less-organised way (e.g., as a single file with all articles stored together, indistinguishable in terms of newspaper, date of publication, and so on).

3.2.2 Preparing Texts for Corpus Analysis

Along with attending to theoretical considerations, Brookes and Baker (2021) also had to take into account some practical considerations when designing and building their corpus. In this case, the news texts they downloaded from

LexisNexis required processing prior to analysis; otherwise they would contain features which can adversely influence the accuracy of analytical procedures.

One such issue, and one that frequently arises in the compilation of corpora of online resources, relates to the presence of so-called boilerplate text. This refers to language that occurs within a text, but which is likely to constitute 'noise' in the context of an analysis. When downloading news articles from LexisNexis, the text files will include labels which indicate, inter alia, the 'headline', 'byline' and the author's name. As such elements occur in every text in the corpus, these can accumulate quickly and thus become problematic for frequency-based analytical measures. In this case, the researchers could rely on the technical support of Andrew Hardie, also working within the Centre for Corpus Approaches to Social Science (CASS), who repurposed these elements as metadata for storing and searching the corpus on the online corpus query processor CQPweb (Hardie, 2012), while rendering such information in a way that would not interfere with corpus querying procedures. Alternatively, they could have used something like the 'boilerplate removal' function of WordSmith Tools (Scott, 2016), which is also much faster than manually removing boilerplate text by hand. Of course, deciding on what counts as 'boilerplate' material is a subjective judgement which has to be made by the researcher and will depend on the aims of the research.

Another practical issue that Brookes and Baker (2021) had to deal with, and one which can be particularly troublesome during the collection of news texts from archives, was the presence of duplicate material. The LexisNexis database can store multiple versions of a single news text (e.g., the online and print versions of an article). This issue was exacerbated further in the case of online articles which reported on developing news stories. This is because such articles constitute 'live' news texts which are typically updated throughout the day as the story develops or corrections to the original story are made. With each update, a 'new' article is essentially produced, and the original article and all subsequent updates were stored as separate texts in LexisNexis. Like boilerplate text, duplicated material can skew the results of frequency-based analytical techniques while also hindering the representativeness of the corpus in a more general sense.

There are a series of steps through which duplicate texts in a corpus can be identified; first, Brookes and Baker (2021) noticed a large number of duplicated articles by manually reviewing chronologically ordered concordance lines. This prompted the second stage, which was to search for long n-grams (e.g., of seven or more words) automatically, using the corpus analysis tool. N-grams of this length typically occur due to the presence of either quoted material or duplicated articles. Third, the authors searched more systematically for such duplicated material using the 'duplicate text' function within version 7 of WordSmith Tools (Scott, 2016). This function allows users to group the texts within a corpus according to a user-determined threshold of linguistic similarity and then manually check and, if they wish, remove high-similarity results. On the whole, this approach was effective for Brookes and Baker (2021); however, there is no entirely reliable automated way of identifying and removing duplicate texts, and manual checking at each stage is advised. Moreover, like the identification of boilerplate material, deciding on what counts as a duplicate text is up to the corpus compiler and will depend on the aims of the research. For example, to allow for the presence of the repeated use of press copy by the different news providers represented in their corpus (PA Media, Thomson Reuters, United Press International), Brookes and Baker (2021) only searched for and removed duplicated texts *within* newspapers (including online, Sunday and 'sister' editions), rather than looking across newspapers.

This example, from Brookes and Baker, provides some key considerations for building a new corpus of texts that have not been necessarily created for linguistic research. In the next section, we discuss how researchers might adapt texts that have been collected for research purposes, though not originally conceptualised as corpus data.

3.3 Working with Pre-existing Transcript Data from Healthcare Settings

Health communication data can be difficult to collect, and researchers have taken opportunities to use existing datasets for conducting additional analyses of the data collected for a prior study. Two of the reported benefits of this type of secondary analysis include (i) overcoming some of the practical restrictions and resource costs associated with carrying out new data collection and (ii) maximising the value of research that has already been collected (Ruggiano and Perry, 2019). Given that much health communication research is necessarily interdisciplinary, there is also a high probability that datasets are investigated for multiple kinds of analysis. However, data collection will likely be conducted according to specific research practices, reflecting the conventions of the field in which the respective contributors work, and this may deviate from what other collaborators on a project are used to. Even within linguistics, there are different ways of working which shape the fundamental elements of research design, such as how data is collected and how it is documented.

The second case study in this chapter focuses on an international collaboration investigating the interactions that take place in Australian Emergency Departments and, specifically, the work involved in operationalising a collection of transcripts as a corpus. In this example, the researchers were given access to a dataset that was intended for manual qualitative analysis and, subsequently, were tasked with reformatting the data for use with modern corpus analysis software. As a result, we offer some guidance on preparing transcripts that can subsequently be used as corpus files, based on what was involved in this reformatting process.

3.3.1 Communication in Emergency Departments

The data analysed in this case comes from Emergency Department (ED) interactions in Australian hospitals and was collected by a team led by Professor Diana Slade from the Institute for Communication in Health Care (ICH), based at Australia National University. The data was collected for the purposes of a study combining 'discourse analysis of authentic interactions between clinicians and patients; and qualitative ethnographic analysis of the social, organisational, and interdisciplinary clinician practices of each department' (Slade et al., 2015: 11).

EDs are a high-stakes interactional health context in which effective communication can result in life-changing outcomes for patients. There is a clear contribution to be made by linguists in helping to ensure that such communication is effective and supports both the health practitioners in carrying out their care duties and the patients in clearly communicating their needs so that they can be met. Accessing authentic ED interactions is difficult, given the urgency of the encounters and the highly sensitive nature of the personal experiences being discussed. Slade and colleagues (2015: 1–2) summarise what they collected as

> communication between patients and clinicians (doctors, nurses and allied health professionals) in five representative emergency departments in New South Wales and the Australian Capital Territory. The study involved 1093 h of observations, 150 interviews with clinicians and patients, and the audio recording of patient-clinician interactions over the course of 82 patients' emergency department trajectories from triage to disposition.

The dataset therefore represents 'one of the most comprehensive studies internationally on patient-clinician communication in hospitals' (Slade et al., 2015: 2). The original research team produced invaluable analyses of the data from a discourse-analytic approach, which they reported in their book *Communicating in Hospital Emergency Departments* (Slade et al., 2015). What the ICH team collected certainly constitutes an amount of data that is appropriate to benefit from the procedures of corpus analysis and so seemed fitting for secondary analysis using such tools.

3.3.2 Data Transfer

The process of sharing data can introduce challenges that affect what is available to researchers conducting secondary analysis. For instance, there may be ethical concerns if the original consent provided by participants did not account for extending access to the data to those beyond the original research team. Anonymisation may be required before the data is shared, which means that some details may be missing at subsequent stages of analysis.

The ICH team conducted observations and interviews with clinicians and patients, though researchers at CASS have only worked (so far) with the observations that were documented as 'patient journeys' – that is, the full range of interactions that patients experienced from the moment that they entered the ED until their departure or admission into hospital. This large-scale project generated numerous files (audio recordings, researcher notes, information sheets, transcripts, etc.), and the ICH team was able to share their documents with the CASS team in an anonymised form (which precluded the sharing of audio files). However, while the ICH team refers to 82 patient journeys, following the transfer of all associated documents and files, researchers at the CASS Centre were able to identify only 72 patient journey transcripts. This demonstrates one of the potential pitfalls of managing and transferring large datasets.

3.3.3 Data Conversion

The ICH team provided word-processed transcripts of the audio-recorded content captured through their observations of the ED encounters. The transcripts were accompanied by metadata about each participant (i.e., role, gender, age, language background, and nationality), and each transcript included a header with information about the context of the 'patient journey' (presenting illness, diagnosis, duration of visit, triage level, number of health professionals seen, and researcher notes), as shown in Figure 3.1.

The process of creating a corpus from this collection of documents involved reformatting the spoken content as plain text and the additional transcriber notes and other non-speech material as annotation using eXtensible Markup Language (XML), which can be computed by corpus analysis tools such as CQPweb (Hardie, 2012) to carry out tokenisation, lemmatisation, part-of-speech (POS) tagging, and semantic tagging.

While it is a common practice in studies of spoken communication to produce a written version, providing researchers with a tangible record that they can analyse and publish in conventional forms of dissemination (which are primarily typed), transcription is inherently a process of recontextualisation and involves decision-making regarding what is documented and how. Not all aspects will be of relevance to the research, resulting in a variety of transcription systems (Richardson et al., 2023: 5). Alongside spoken content, Sperberg-McQueen and Burnard (1994: 250) remind us that 'the production and comprehension of speech are intimately bound up with the situation in which speech occurs',

3 Collecting Data

Emergency Communication – Hospital P	
Data Information	
Patient number	P017 - Denae
Transcript number	1
Recording date	25 September 2007
Sound file number	070925P017a&bP (two files)
Recorded by	
Move Analysis	

Background Information Patient			
Gender: Female	DOB:	Ethnicity: Anglo	Language: English
Presenting concern:	Fracture – left foot injury		
Triage number: 4	Time arrived: 13:45		
Time Triaged: 14:30		Time 1st seen by Dr: 15:30	
Time Left ED: 16:07		Total Time in ED: 1 hr 37mins	
Other information			

Background Information Health Practitioner/s			
Health Practitioner1	Triage Nurse		
Gender: Female	Age:	Ethnicity:	Language: English
Other information			
Health Practitioner2	Doctor		
Gender: Female	Age:	Ethnicity:	Language: NESB
Other information	RMO or Registrar?		

Transcript

Key to participants	P	Patient
	N	Nurse (triage)
	Z1	Unidentified female staff member
	R1	Researcher
	D	Doctor
	R2	Researcher

Sound file: 070925P017aP

Interactive Structure	Turns/Moves	Speaker	Text
		P	…pain, it's been two weeks.
		N	Okay. = = So …
		P	= = So anyway, that's …
		N	And that's – and which ankle are we = = talking

P017 – Denae

Figure 3.1 The first page of a transcript document.

prompting us to incorporate contextual features when we document speech. However, they also assert that 'determining which are relevant is not always simple' (1994: 250). Furthermore, if the researcher plans to investigate the

3.3 Pre-existing Transcript Data from Healthcare Settings

frequency and distribution of such features using corpus tools, they need to be encoded in a format that lends itself to corpus query.

Slade and colleagues (2015: xi) produced orthographic transcripts, favouring standard English spelling but using non-standard forms to capture 'idiosyncratic or dialectal pronunciations (e.g., gonna)'. They refer to fillers and hesitation markers, which were 'transcribed as they are spoken, using the standard English variants (e.g., ah, uh huh, hmm and mmm)' (2015: xi). Finally, they explain that punctuation marks were broadly used according to their meaning 'in standard written English', though also used to indicate additional special meaning, such as putting words in parentheses when the content was unclear and according to 'the transcriber's best analysis' (Slade et al., 2015: xi). Slade and colleagues' (2015) notation system is consistent with wider transcription practices in the field (see Sperberg-McQueen and Burnard, 1994; Fraser, 2022) and demonstrates the influence of the system outlined by Jefferson (2004), which is widely used across the social sciences and strongly associated with conversation analysis. As such, the transcription system aligns with the analytical procedures that the ICH team was to carry out.

We can, however, begin to see potential issues in the transcript notation demonstrated in Jefferson (2004) for corpus tools that rely on computing regular forms. For instance, the Jeffersonian system suggests using parenthesized 'h' to indicate plosiveness (i.e., s(h)orr(h)y). This vocal quality can result from high emotional states, such as crying or laughter, as well as difficulties producing speech because of physical discomfort – all of which would be likely and pertinent in a study of patients in hospital EDs. However, this variant form would not be included in a simple corpus query for 'sorry', which may be an unintended consequence. As an alternative that would also facilitate the automatic conversion to a 'corpus-ready' format, a transcriber could record this as 'sorry [#heavy breathing]'.

Collins and Hardie (2022) summarised the main tasks required in the conversion of the transcript documents to corpus files, and developed recommendations for a transcript notation system that would serve to optimise this process in the future. Collins and Hardie's (2022: 132) recommendations are largely designed 'to generate minimal ambiguity when qualitative-research transcription data is mapped to XML or other structured format and operationalised as a searchable corpus'. An example from the ED data of the kind of ambiguity that such recommendations were created to address comes with the transcriber's use of square brackets, which were used for the following purposes:

- Redacting personal information: 'My name is [patient name].'
- Embedded turns: 'I know it coming, the phlegm black. [D Mm mm] No more.'
- Describing contextual features: [background noise]

The alternative suggested by Collins and Hardie (2022: 131) is to indicate different uses of square brackets using a flag character:

- Vocalisation: [@laughs]
- Transcriber comment: [#D fills in form]
- Embedded utterance: [=P yeah]
- Redaction: [name]

This minor adjustment to existing practice will not impede manual analysis but does make it entirely mechanistic to automatically convert the above to XML or another structured format, as follows:

- [@laughs] becomes <voc desc="laughs"/>
- [#D fills in form] becomes <comment content="D fills in form"/>
- [=P yeah] becomes <u who="P" trans="overlap">yeah</u>
- [name] becomes <anon type="person"/>

The designation and function of such flag characters can be adapted to the different levels of specification required for the study.

An extract of one of the transcripts is shown in Table 3.2, and the CASS team was able to use this tabulated format to automatically extract speaker information and spoken content, applying additional scripts to retain the non-speech material that also appeared in the rows in the column (sometimes marked with different formatting; e.g., bold font).

We can see in Table 3.2 how the rows of the table align the spoken material (and sometimes other contextual information) with a speaker ID, and when combined with the case file (i.e., the specific patient journey), this creates a unique speaker identifier (P27_D2), which was recorded in XML as follows:

<u who=P27D2>And they said you had a little bit of (.) blockage there but nothing too exciting?</u>

This example shows the introduction of utterance boundaries, marked at the beginning (with additional speaker information) and the end, with each cell in

Table 3.2 *Extract of a transcript in the Emergency Department corpus*

Speaker	Text
D2	And you had an angiogram eight years ago was it?
P	Mm, something like that.
D2	And they said you had a little bit of ... blockage there but nothing too exciting?
P	Well they – because the blockage was close to a branch ...
D2	Yes.
P	Ah, the surgeon said no, it's too dangerous to operate. (background noise)

3.3 Pre-existing Transcript Data from Healthcare Settings

the 'Text' column, as shown in Table 3.2, approximately mapped onto a speaker turn or utterance. Establishing utterance boundaries and linking these to speakers enabled the research team to subsequently carry out restricted queries and target speakers according to their metadata (e.g., only content provided by doctors and/or female speakers and/or speakers, aged 30–34). This restricted query functionality was used by Collins and co-authors (2022) to investigate the frequency and type of questioning utterances as they were produced by doctors according to different levels of seniority. Finally, the CASS team was able to refer to the transcript notation (with additional manual checking) to separate contextual information and non-speech material from the content in the 'Text' cells and convert them to a format that would exclude them from token counts and content queries, as follows:

<event desc="background noise"/>

Figure 3.2 demonstrates how the extract appeared, following conversion, in the extended context view of CQPweb. This includes the reformatting of pauses to minimise the potential ambiguity of using ellipses, '(. . .)', by using the alternative, more clearly defined notation '(.)'.

As shown earlier in Figure 3.1, the metadata associated with each patient journey was also documented according to a template. The ICH team, however, was working in highly dynamic environments, striving to minimise the disruption to the natural flow of events caused by their presence. As such, as is the case with most large-scale data-collection studies, some details were not recorded and there is variability in the form of the metadata that was collected. For instance, participant ages were indicated to different levels of specificity ('22', 'mid-30s', 'young') and based on the researcher's approximation. The CASS team thus devised a regularised categorisation scheme for age (i.e., 18–24, 25–29, 30–4,

P27_D2: And you had an angiogram eight years ago was it ?

P27_P: Mm , something like that .

P27_D2: And they said you had a little bit of (.) blockage there but nothing too exciting ?

P27_P: Well they - because the blockage was close to a branch

(.) **P27_D2:** Yes .

P27_P: Ah , the surgeon said no , it 's too dangerous to operate .

(background noise)

Figure 3.2 A passage of the transcript as it appears in the extended context view of CQPweb.

35–9, etc.) and other metadata that allowed us to retain a large portion of the recorded information while also supporting combinations of restricted corpus queries (e.g., selecting 30–4 and 35–9 would facilitate a search of content produced by speakers in their thirties).

We recommend comprehensively documenting contextual information for current and future research projects. However, researchers may be working with data which was produced and archived in the past and for which such information needs to be recovered. In the next section, we discuss what this can involve for corpus compilation.

3.4 Building a Historical Corpus of Anti-vaccination Literature

Our final example in this chapter involves building a corpus of historical texts, specifically the Victorian Anti-Vaccination Discourse Corpus (VicVaDis), which was briefly introduced in Chapter 1 and is discussed by Hardaker and colleagues (2024). In this section we describe what motivated the creation of this corpus and the process that led to its completion. We discuss the decisions that needed to be made along the way, focusing particularly on those that apply to the building of historical corpora. In contrast with the examples presented in the previous two sections, the team who created the VicVaDis corpus (Hardaker et al., 2024) did not initially know whether enough relevant texts had survived from the Victorian period to create a dataset large enough to benefit from the use of corpus methods. Even when the researchers established that a reasonable number of texts were indeed available and convertible to machine-readable format, it was impossible to be certain about how representative those texts might be of the totality of relevant texts from the period, because many, or perhaps most, have not survived until the present day. These issues are also likely to apply to the creation of historical corpora more generally, including from different periods and on different topics.

3.4.1 Vaccine Hesitancy in History

We begin with the motivation for building the VicVaDis corpus. Vaccinations are well known to be the focus of present-day controversies. On the one hand, they are deemed to be one of the most effective public health tools and have made it possible to eradicate or reduce the impact of a wide range of infectious diseases, including smallpox, polio, tetanus, meningitis, yellow fever, measles, Ebola and, most recently, COVID-19 (WHO, 2022). On the other hand, in 2019 the World Health Organization included among the top 10 threats to global health 'vaccine hesitancy', which they defined as 'the reluctance or refusal to vaccinate despite the availability of vaccines' (WHO, 2019). Indeed, vaccine hesitancy has affected vaccination programmes in 90 per cent of countries in

3.4 A Historical Corpus of Anti-vaccination Literature

the world (Lancet, 2019) and was further highlighted as a major public health concern during the COVID-19 pandemic (e.g., Hughes et al., 2021).

The spread of anti-vaccination arguments has also been associated with the internet and the rise of social media (e.g., Nuwarda et al., 2022). However, vaccine hesitancy is not in fact a recent phenomenon and has been a concern for as long as vaccinations have existed (Durbach, 2005). The VicVaDis corpus was built to capture the anti-vaccination movement that arose in the second half of the nineteenth century in England, during the reign of Queen Victoria, when the vaccine against smallpox was made compulsory for babies (Tafuri et al., 2014). Smallpox was highly infectious and had a mortality rate of at least 30 per cent (Stewart and Devlin, 2006). At the end of the eighteenth century, Edward Jenner, an English doctor, built on long-standing folk knowledge to assert that those who had contracted the milder illness cowpox were immune to smallpox. He subsequently introduced the first 'vaccination' (from Latin *vacca*) – that is, the practice of introducing material from the pustules of cowpox sufferers under the skin of a healthy person, causing a reaction that resulted in immunity to smallpox. Jenner is deemed to have saved more lives than any other person in history (Stewart and Devlin, 2006), and following widespread vaccination campaigns, smallpox was declared eradicated by the Thirty-Third World Health Assembly in 1980.

In nineteenth-century England, however, mandates for vaccination and the use of material derived from animals were among the reasons that caused major resistance, manifested, for example, in a demonstration involving around 100,000 people in Leicester in 1885 (Charlton, 1983; Durbach, 2005). For insight into the vaccine-hesitant sentiment at the time, consider the following extracts from 2 of the 133 texts included in the VicVaDis corpus (Hardaker et al., 2024: 169–70):

> In October 1876 an official inquiry was made concerning the illnesses through vaccination of sixteen children in the Misterton district of the Gainsborough Union, of which six proved fatal, but no mention was made of vaccination in any of the *death* certificates. Of the four deaths at Norwich, the subject also of an official inquiry in 1882, only one was certified as being due to vaccination. It appeared that nine children were vaccinated in June by Dr. Guy, the public vaccinator; of these four were dead of erysipelas within three weeks of the operation, and five were seriously ill from constitutional disease. (Tebb, 1889, *What Is the Truth about Vaccination?*)

> A wider, and deeper, and subtler *Social* Evil than universal Compulsory Vaccination is scarcely conceivable; on the physical side, universal pollution; on the side of manhood, womanhood, and childhood, with their several dignities, it is to the extent of its reach, degradation and extinction. The cradle is born to an immediate medical hell. Politically, *Compulsory Vaccination* is an innermost stab of Liberty which piercing its heart, will find its courage and heaven-born principles and convictions in other directions an easy prey. State medicine can do what it likes with us, if we once let it do this. (1879, LSACV, *The Vaccination Inquirer and Health Review: The Organ of the London Society*)

The Victorian anti-vaccination movement has been studied by historians (e.g., Durbach, 2005), but prior to the creation of the VicVaDis corpus, there was no textual dataset that would enable large-scale linguistic studies of the anti-vaccination arguments of the time. The corpus was thus created to make it possible to carry out such studies, in order to complement historical research and to enable comparisons with present-day discussions of vaccinations, which already benefit from the availability of corpora (e.g., Coltman-Patel et al., 2022). As we describe in more detail in the following sections, the VicVaDis corpus contains approximately 3.5 million words, drawn from anti-vaccination texts that would have been widely available to the population at the time.

3.4.2 Creating the Corpus

Hardaker and colleagues (2024) began with a series of exploratory searches of online collections of texts covering the relevant historical period to establish how much textual material was still available on the topic of vaccination. This revealed that a substantial amount of such material still existed, particularly in three specific text archives: (1) the Wellcome Collection Library (https://wellcomecollection.org), (2) Project Gutenberg (www.gutenberg.org), and (3) Online Library of Liberty (https://oll.libertyfund.org). The team used 'vaccination' as a search term to query all three text archives. Among other things, this led to the retrieval of *A Catalogue of Anti-Vaccination Literature*, which was issued by the *London Society for the Abolition of Compulsory Vaccination* (the LSACV). This catalogue, which contains 205 texts, was used to identify any additional documents beyond those retrieved from the initial three archives. This led to more targeted searches in the UK Medical Heritage Library (UKMHL, www.medicalheritage.org), the British Library Nineteenth-Century Collection (www.bl.uk), JSTOR (www.jstor.org), and the Internet Archive (https://archive.org).[2] Once these documents were retrieved, the criteria for including them in the corpus concerned topic, time, location, genre, and technical quality.

With regard to topic, the team only included texts that took an anti-vaccination stance. This was established by considering titles (e.g., *The Evils of Vaccination: With a Protest against Its Legal Enforcement*), consulting sources (e.g., the

---

[2] These resources linked to documents in the following further archives: the US National Library of Medicine, Bristol Selected Pamphlets, the London School of Economics Selected Pamphlets, the Francis A. Countway Library of Medicine, the Harold B. Lee Library, the London School of Hygiene and Tropical Medicine Library and Archives Service, the Royal College of Physicians in Edinburgh, the Royal College of Surgeons of England, and the online collections of Harvard University, Oxford University, Saint Mary's College of California, University of California, University of Glasgow, University of Leeds, and the Cushing/Whitney Medical Library at Yale University. In addition, some documents were uploaded by private individuals to the Internet Archive.

3.4 A Historical Corpus of Anti-vaccination Literature

London Society for the Abolition of Compulsory Vaccination) and, where necessary, becoming familiar with the texts themselves.

With regard to time period, the team considered the dates of the seven vaccination acts that were passed by Parliament in England with regard to the smallpox vaccine. The first such act dated from 1840, but it was the 1853 act that made mandatory the vaccination of babies by the age of three months, with the introduction of fines and imprisonment for parents who did not comply. Four subsequent acts introduced various changes in legislation but did not substantially change the mandatory nature of vaccination. This changed with the 1907 Vaccination Act (shortly after the end of Queen Victoria's reign), which made it relatively easy for parents to opt out of vaccination without incurring penalties. This effectively marked the end of compulsory smallpox vaccination. Against this background, it was decided that the VicVaDis corpus would include documents published between 1854 and 1906.

With regard to place of publication, the researchers were interested in documents from England and Wales, where the vaccination acts applied. However, no documents published in Wales were retrieved from the various archives. Therefore, the VicVaDis corpus includes only texts published in England.

With regard to genre, the searches posed by Hardaker and colleagues identified a wide variety of types of texts that could be considered for inclusion:

- Pamphlets and popular journals produced by anti-vaccination campaigners
- Local newspaper reports and letters to local newspapers
- Papers presented to Parliament by John Simon in 1857 (e.g., cited by Williamson, 2007; Durbach, 2005)
- Letters from prominent doctors to various public bodies and publications
- Medical journals: *The Lancet* and the *BMJ* (analysed by Kondrlik, 2020)
- A summary of positions on vaccination in the *Edinburgh Review* (1810), a leading political and literary magazine (analysed by Williamson, 2007)
- Materials gathered in the *Monthly Review*, which predated the *Edinburgh Review*, aimed at non-specialist but educated readers (analysed by Arnold & Arnold, 2022)
- Contemporary medical histories and textbooks (Hardaker et al., 2024: 165)

While this variety of texts was available for inclusion, the researchers' primary interest was in non-fictional texts that were aimed for and accessible to the general public, namely pamphlets, newsletters, non-academic tracts and periodicals, and letters to newspapers. The corpus thus excludes fiction and drama, and legal, scientific, and medical publications. The reasons for this decision were as follows: Although literacy rates in England and Wales increased rapidly during the nineteenth century, specialist texts aimed for expert educated audiences had limited circulation, due to a combination of cost and venue of publication. They are also the texts that tend to be relied upon in existing historical studies. In contrast, more 'popular' texts have not been extensively studied but were in fact widely available to people at the time. Pamphlets, for example, were produced quickly and distributed cheaply or free of charge (Humphries, 2011). As such, the material included in the corpus can be seen as the closest equivalent at the time of today's posts on social media.

With regard to technical quality, inclusion was based on the success rates of employing optical character recognition (OCR) software to convert the documents retrieved – mostly as PDFs – from the archives into a plain text format that could be processed by (corpus) software tools. Having tested the quality of different OCR tools, the conversion process was carried out via Adobe Acrobat, and a tailor-made Perl script was employed to identify words in the converted documents that included non-alphabetic characters, such as numbers and punctuation. A quality threshold of 70 per cent accuracy was then adopted as a criterion for inclusion in the corpus. In other words, documents with scores of less than 70 per cent were excluded. This was regarded as an adequate reflection of the error rate in the process of conversion.

Finally, in contrast with the creation of many other types of corpora, the VicVaDis corpus did not pose any issues of ethics and copyright. All relevant documents were in the public domain, and any copyright restrictions had long expired.

3.4.3 The VicVaDis Corpus

The VicVaDis corpus consists of 133 texts and 3,488,959 tokens calculated using the corpus analysis toolkit AntConc (Anthony, 2023). Texts vary considerably in length. The shortest is a 195-word letter to the *East London Observer* from 1985. The longest is *The Anti-Vaccinator and Public Health Journal 1872–3*, a 362,864-word anthology edited by John Pickering which includes letters, notes, public addresses, and reports. The texts involve 66 unique declared authorship designations. These include not just named individuals but also, for example, anonyms and pseudonyms (e.g., *A Sufferer*) and organisations (e.g., the LSACV).

The chronological dispersion of documents in VicVaDis is shown in Figure 3.3 (Hardaker et al., 2024: 7).

The mean number of texts per year is 2.5, but as Figure 3.3 shows, the number of texts per year varies, with no texts in some years and peaks in others (e.g., 11 documents in 1889). However, we should not necessarily consider the peaks and troughs as a reflection of the number of anti-vaccination documents published in different years. Rather, these figures are largely dependent on what was retrievable from the various archives, and on the error rate that resulted from OCR conversion.

Overall, for historical corpora such as the VicVaDis corpus, it is particularly difficult to reach the standards of representativeness and balance

3.4 A Historical Corpus of Anti-vaccination Literature

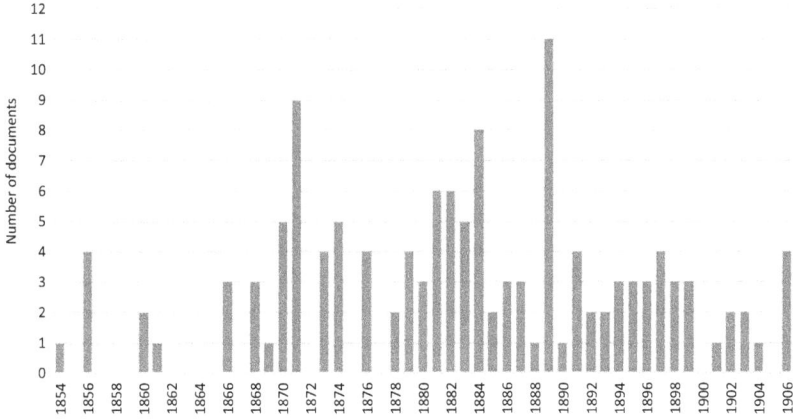

Figure 3.3 Chronological dispersion of texts in the VicVaDis corpus.

that are achievable in the creation of present-day corpora, such as the news corpus on obesity described earlier in this chapter. Hardaker and colleagues (2024) explained this as follows:

As in any corpus, there is a tension between the human-imposed notion of *balance* across, for instance, authors, texts, dates, and so forth, and the more organic principle of *representativeness*.... Even in contemporary corpora, objective representativeness is generally an ideal, and in historical corpora such a goal is less achievable still, given the fundamental lack of ground truth. In our case, we have no way of identifying all of the anti-vaccination literature in circulation throughout the 53 years that our texts cover, and some – or possibly, most – of it will be lost without trace. We therefore have no rigorous benchmarks against which to measure our corpus and so cannot know whether particular years, authors, or texts are over- or under-represented. (Hardaker et al., 2024: 167)

It may in fact be possible to add further texts to the corpus if more documents are retrieved in the future and/or if improvements in the success rates of OCR conversion bring more documents above the 70 per cent technical quality threshold. Nonetheless, as shown in Hardaker and colleagues (2024), even with its inevitable limitations, the VicVaDis corpus constitutes an important resource for the study of anti-vaccination arguments in the Victorian period, and for diachronic or cross-cultural comparisons of vaccination-related discourses. The corpus is freely available through the UK Data Service (https://reshare.ukdataservice.ac.uk/856736/).

3.5 Conclusion

Researchers are tasked with making a number of decisions when it comes to collecting data, and corpus linguists typically have to reconcile the theoretical principles of good corpus design with the practical challenges of data availability. The resources through which we access our data can be very influential in shaping the corpus that we eventually compile, both in terms of what is included in a data archive, for example, and the quality of the content and associated metadata. What we have shown through the case studies discussed in this chapter is that however we come to collect our data, there are certain steps that we can take to optimise the utility of our corpus for systematic and rigorous analysis. For instance, we can reduce the 'noise' of our investigations of health discourses by removing 'boilerplate' text, and we can make sure that our interpretations are informed by contextual factors by recording salient metadata. Taking the time to pre-process the data, for example, in applying annotation for paralinguistic features or regularising spelling, can also be beneficial for enabling researchers to query these features. Ultimately, familiarising oneself with the characteristics of the data and the capabilities of the corpus software tools can ensure that researchers are able to get the most out of the data.

References

Anthony, L. (2023). *AntConc* (Version 4.2.4) [Computer Software]. Waseda University. Available from www.laurenceanthony.net/software.

Arnold, W. and Arnold, C. (2022). Medicine in the *Monthly Review*: Revealing Public Medical Discourse through Topic Modelling. *Digital Scholarship in the Humanities, 37*(3), 611–29. https://doi.org/10.1093/llc/fqab034.

Baker, P. (2009). The BE06 Corpus of British English and Recent Language Change. *International Journal of Corpus Linguistics, 14*(3), 312–37. https://doi.org/10.1075/ijcl.14.3.02bak.

Biber, D. (1993). Representativeness in Corpus Design. *Literary and Linguistic Computing, 8*(4), 243–57. https://doi.org/10.1093/llc/8.4.243.

(2004). Representativeness in Corpus Design. In G. Sampson and D. McCarthy (eds.), *Corpus Linguistics: Readings in a Widening Perspective* (pp. 174–97). Continuum.

Brookes, G. (2023). Killer, Thief or Companion? A Corpus-Based Study of Dementia Metaphors in UK Tabloids. *Metaphor and Symbol, 38*(3), 213–30. https://doi.org/10.1080/10926488.2022.2142472.

Brookes, G. and Baker, P. (2021). *Obesity in the News: Language and Representation in the British Press*. Cambridge University Press.

Charlton C. (1983). The Fight against Vaccination: The Leicester Demonstration of 1885. *Local Population Studies, 30*, 60–6. Available at www.localpopulationstudies.org.uk/PDF/LPS30/LPS30_1983_60–66.pdf.

Collins, L. C., Gablasova, D. and Pill, J. (2022). 'Doing Questioning' in the Emergency Department (ED). *Health Communication*, *38*(12), 2721–9. https://doi.org/10.10 80/10410236.2022.2111630.

Collins, L. C. and Hardie, A. (2022). Making Use of Transcription Data from Qualitative Research within a Corpus-Linguistic Paradigm: Issues, Experiences and Recommendations. *Corpora*, *17*(1), 123–35. https://doi.org/10.3366/cor.2022.0237.

Coltman-Patel, T., Dance, W., Demjén, Z., Gatherer, D., Hardaker, C. and Semino, E. (2022). 'Am I Being Unreasonable to Vaccinate My Kids against My Ex's Wishes?' – A Corpus Linguistic Exploration of Conflict in Vaccination Discussions on Mumsnet Talk's AIBU Forum. *Discourse, Context & Media*, *48*, 100624. https://doi.org/10.1016/j.dcm.2022.100624.

Durbach, N. (2005). *Bodily Matters: The Anti-Vaccination Movement in England, 1853–1907*. Duke University Press.

Fraser, H. (2022). A Framework for Deciding How to Create and Evaluate Transcripts for Forensic and Other Purposes. *Frontiers in Communication*, *7*, 898410. https://doi.org/10.3389/fcomm.2022.898410.

Hardaker, C., Deignan, A., Semino, E., Coltman-Patel, T., Dance, W., Demjén, Z., Sanderson, C. and Gatherer, D. (2024). The Victorian Anti-Vaccination Discourse Corpus (VicVaDis): Construction and Exploration. *Digital Scholarship in the Humanities*, *39*, 162–74. https://doi.org/10.1093/llc/fqad075.

Hardie, A. (2012). CQPweb – Combining Power, Flexibility and Usability in a Corpus Analysis Tool. *International Journal of Corpus Linguistics*, *17*(3), 380–409. https://doi.org/10.1075/ijcl.17.3.04har.

  (2014). Modest XML for Corpora: Not a Standard, but a Suggestion. *ICAME Journal*, *38*(1), 73–103. https://doi.org/10.2478/icame-2014-0004.

Hughes, B., Miller-Idriss, C., Piltch-Loeb, R., Goldberg, B., White, K., Criezis, M. and Savoia, E. (2021). Development of a Codebook of Online Anti-Vaccination Rhetoric to Manage COVID-19 Vaccine Misinformation. *International Journal of Environmental Research and Public Health*, *18*(14), 7556. www.mdpi.com/1660-4601/18/14/7556.

Humphries, B. (2011). Nineteenth Century Pamphlets Online. *The Ephemerist*, 153. The Ephemera Society. Available at http://eprints.lse.ac.uk/40202/.

Jefferson, G. (2004). Glossary of Transcript Symbols with an Introduction. In G. Lerner (ed.), *Conversation Analysis: Studies from the First Generation* (pp. 13–31). John Benjamins. https://doi.org/10.1075/pbns.125.02jef.

Kondrlik, K. E. (2020). Conscientious Objection to Vaccination and the Failure to Solidify Professional Identity in Late Victorian Socio-Medical Journals. *Victorian Periodicals Review*, *53*(3), 338–71. https://doi.org/10.1353/vpr.2020.0032.

The Lancet Child & Adolescent Health. (2019). Vaccine Hesitancy: A Generation at Risk. *The Lancet Child & Adolescent Health*, *3*(5), 281. https://doi.org/10.1016/S2352-4642(19)30092-6.

McEnery, T. and Hardie, A. (2012). *Corpus Linguistics: Method, Theory and Practice*. Cambridge University Press.

Nuwarda, R. F., Ramzan, I., Weekes, L. and Kayser, V. (2022). Vaccine Hesitancy: Contemporary Issues and Historical Background. *Vaccines*, *10*(10), 1595. https://doi.org/10.3390/vaccines10101595.

Rayson, P. (2008). From Key Words to Key Semantic Domains. *International Journal of Corpus Linguistics*, *13*(4), 519–49. https://doi.org/10.1075/ijcl.13.4.06ray.

Reppen, R. (2022). Building a Corpus: What Are Key Considerations? In A. O'Keeffe and M. J. McCarthy (eds.), *The Routledge Handbook of Corpus Linguistics*, 2nd ed. (pp. 13–20). Routledge. https://doi.org/10.4324/9780367076399-2.

Richardson, E., Hamann, M., Tompkinson, J., Haworth, K. and Deamer, F. (2023). Understanding the Role of Transcription in Evidential Consistency of Police Interview Records in England and Wales. *Language in Society*. Online first. 1–32. https://doi.org/10.1017/S004740452300060X.

Ruggiano, N. and Perry, T. E. (2019). Conducting Secondary Analysis of Qualitative Data: Should We, Can We, and How? *Qualitative Social Work*, *18*(1), 81–97. https://doi.org/10.1177/1473325017700701.

Scott, M. (2016). *WordSmith Tools* (version 7). Lexical Analysis Software.

(2017). *News Downloads and Aboutness*. Plenary speech at the International Corpus Linguistics conference. Birmingham: University of Birmingham. 26 July 2017. www.youtube.com/watch?v=3FVa0KwtvLc.

Scott, M. and Tribble, C. (2006). *Key Words and Corpus Analysis in Language Education*. John Benjamins.

Slade, D., Manidis, M., McGregor, J., Scheeres, H., Chandler, E., Stein-Parbury, J., Dunston, R., Herke, M. and Matthiessen, C. M. I. M. (2015). *Communicating in Hospital Emergency Departments*. Springer.

Sperberg-McQueen, C. and Burnard, L. (1994). *Guidelines for Electronic Text Encoding and Interchange (TEI P3). Text Encoding Initiative*. https://tei-c.org/Vault/GL/P4beta.pdf.

Stewart, A. J. and Devlin, P. M. (2006). The History of the Smallpox Vaccine. *Journal of Infection*, *52*(5), 329–34. https://doi.org/10.1016/j.jinf.2005.07.021.

Tafuri, S., Gallone, M. S., Cappelli, M. G., Martinelli, D., Prato, R. and Germinario, C. (2014). Addressing the Anti-Vaccination Movement and the Role of HCWs. *Vaccine*, *32*(38), 4860–5. https://doi.org/10.1016/j.vaccine.2013.11.006.

Williamson, S. (2007). *The Vaccination Controversy: The Rise, Reign and Fall of Compulsory Vaccination for Smallpox*. Liverpool University Press.

World Health Organization (WHO) (2019). Top Ten Threats to Global Health in 2019. www.who.int/news-room/spotlight/ten-threats-to-global-health-in-2019.

(2022). Vaccines and Immunization. www.who.int/health-topics/vaccines-and-immunization.

4 Ethics

4.1 Introduction

Issues that need to be considered when planning to conduct a linguistic study include the ethical implications of collecting and analysing data, the institutional requirements placed on the project and any legal requirements relevant to the proposed work. When the study involves a corpus, the aim of collecting, analysing and quoting from large amounts of data can give rise to difficult questions. Do we need to gain permission from every person involved in creating each text in a corpus? Should we anonymise all references to names and identities across millions of words of text? Is there any point in making a corpus text anonymous when a version of it may exist online which can easily be retrieved with a search tool?

In this chapter we begin with an overview of the ethical aspects of creating corpora from different kinds of data sources relevant to health(care) and then focus on two studies that involved different approaches to addressing ethical issues.

Broadly speaking, ethics in the context of research involves ensuring that no harm is caused to people when conducting a study. In healthcare research, harm does not just include negative physical consequences, as may be caused, for example, when testing a new drug. It may also include potential psychological and social harm (Demjén et al., 2023: 37).

For example, reporting or quoting from interviews or online forum posts can potentially lead to a loss of privacy or anonymity for the people involved, which can in turn cause distress, damage social relationships and reduce people's willingness to engage with healthcare services.

In healthcare research, three main considerations, known as the 'Belmont Principles', are widely applied to protect the people involved in the research (Beauchamp and Childress, 2001): the first is respect for persons, the second is beneficence and the third is justice. Respect for persons involves treating people as autonomous agents and protecting anybody who may have reduced autonomy (e.g., children or prisoners). Beneficence involves avoiding harm to people and, as much as possible, maximising their well-being. Justice involves treating people equitably and making sure that the research benefits the groups who most need or are entitled to be benefited.

Different types of data and analyses in corpus-based research on health and illness pose different degrees and kinds of ethical concerns. This will affect whether you need to apply to a relevant research ethics committee for approval for your study, and the complexity of the process involved (for a more detailed overview, see Demjén et al., 2023: 38ff.).

Minimal ethical issues are normally posed by material that is in the public domain and that was produced for wide audiences by people working in a professional capacity. This includes news reports, policy documents, websites of health-related organisations and so on. Historical materials, such as the nineteenth-century anti-vaccination literature described in Chapter 3, also fall into this category. While ethics approval from a relevant institutional committee may still be required to collect and analyse the data, the risk of any harm arising from the research is very low.

In contrast, major ethical issues, in contrast, are posed by material collected from private and confidential communicative settings involving individuals and their personal lives. This includes, for example, letters from consultants to patients and any recording of interactions between patients and healthcare professionals. In such cases the risks to patients in terms of loss of privacy and anonymity are very high, and obtaining ethics approval from the relevant bodies is likely to be a lengthy and complex process. As interactions from healthcare settings are also often time-consuming to collect, corpus-based studies of such material are rare. An exception is the study of a large corpus of transcripts of Emergency Department interactions discussed in Chapter 3.

User-generated content from social media platforms and online forums tends to fall somewhere in the middle with regard to ethical issues, depending on a variety of factors. In the next section, we consider health-related online forums specifically and explain how access and ethics approval were obtained for the purposes of a corpus-based study of online interactions about the experience of pain.

4.2 Ethical Considerations When Studying Online Forums: Research on a Forum Dedicated to Pain

Health-related online forums can play an important part in people's experience of illness, as they make it possible to discuss one's condition and concerns with others who share similar experiences while remaining anonymous. Anonymity in online interactions is associated with what Suler (2004) calls a 'disinhibition effect' and can be exploited for the purposes of spreading disinformation or creating conflict (Graham and Hardaker, 2017). However, anonymous online environments also make it possible for people to (i) share experiences that are

4.2 Ethical Considerations When Studying Online Forums

too private or harrowing to discuss with family and friends; (ii) give and receive honest and disinterested information, advice and support; and (iii) create valuable bonds that improve people's quality of life and make it easier to cope with the difficulties associated with illness (Eysenbach et al., 2004; Smith-Merry et al., 2019; Yip, 2020).

Interactions on online forums can be studied from a variety of disciplinary perspectives and by means of different qualitative and quantitative methods. Among these, corpus methods are particularly relevant, as online forums are typically are typically sources of large volumes of machine readable text. Analysing those texts systematically usually requires the ability to handle millions of words of data. On the other hand, the collection of large quantities of data from online forums makes it difficult, or even potentially disruptive to the forum itself, to attempt to obtain consent from individual contributors to collect forum posts for inclusion in a corpus (Hunt and Brookes, 2020: 70ff.). What are the implications of this for planning corpus-based studies of online forums?

4.2.1 Online Forums and Ethics

In order to decide whether and how to conduct a corpus study of online forum data, it is necessary to consider several interacting factors:

- *Access*: does the forum require a members' login to read contributions and to post contributions?
- *Terms and conditions of use*: do participants give consent to their contributions being used for research purposes when they register on the forum and, if so, what is the nature of that consent?
- *Perceptions of privacy*: is there evidence that participants perceive their interactions to be private?
- *Anonymity*: to what extent and how will data collection, analysis and dissemination of results ensure the anonymity of forum contributors?
- *Risk of harm*: to what extent could participants be harmed if their identity were to be (even partially) revealed as a result of the research?
- *Potential benefit*: to what extent and how could participants or other related groups benefit from the research?

In addition to the academic literature (e.g., Mackenzie, 2017; Demjén et al., 2023: 38ff.), guidance on these ethical issues is provided and regularly updated by, for example, the Association of Internet Researchers (Franzke et al., 2020) and the British Association for Applied Linguistics (BAAL, 2021).

In the rest of this section, we present one solution to the ethical issues involved in analysing online forums dedicated to health: obtaining posts written by people who had previously consented for their contributions to the forum to be used for research purposes. Our example involves an online forum dedicated to pain, but the same considerations would apply regardless of the health condition involved.

4.2.2 The Pain Concern Forum

The online forum we consider in this section is called the Pain Concern forum (Collins and Semino, 2024). It is run by the UK-based charity Pain Concern and is hosted by private company HealthUnlocked. Pain Concern advocates for better services and a better understanding of the needs of people living with pain. As part of its activities, it runs a helpline and produces leaflets, a magazine and an internet radio programme. The corpus analysed by Collins and Semino consists of contributions posted on the forum between May 2012 and October 2020, for a total of 89,741 posts and 8,543,729 tokens (token count as retrieved via CQPweb).

The forum is one of more than 300 health-related online communities hosted on the website of HealthUnlocked, whose stated aim is to 'transform individual health experiences into support, insight and understanding for others. We do this by enabling people to share personal health experiences and information online using our site ("Our Site"). In turn this provides support, aids self-management, and improves interactions with professionals, with the aim of improving day-to-day health and well-being' (https://support.healthunlocked .com/article/148-privacy).

With regard to access, posts on HealthUnlocked are only partly public, in that non-members have a restricted view – enough to determine whether they are sufficiently interested to create an account, but not to read all the material posted on any community. Creating an account is free and gives access to all the communities hosted on the site.

As a business, HealthUnlocked operates by selling access to material posted on the site to commercial or research organisations. This is reflected in the terms and conditions for access to the site. When they sign up for an account, users are asked whether they are willing to give permission for their posts to be used for research purposes by HealthUnlocked partners. The preference expressed at first registration can subsequently be changed. The analysis of the Pain Concern online forum was carried out as part of a contractual arrangement between HealthUnlocked and the ESRC Centre for Corpus Approaches to Social Science (CASS) at Lancaster University, which also involved the online forum of the charity Anxiety Support (Collins and Baker, 2023; see Chapters 5, 7, and 9). As part of the contract, the researchers received an anonymised download of contributions from users who had consented to their contributions being used for research purposes at the point when the data was downloaded.

This kind of blanket consent reduces the need to consider the content of contributions for evidence of perceptions of privacy, even though researchers

4.2 Ethical Considerations When Studying Online Forums

should be mindful of this in the analysis. As for anonymity, users create their own usernames as part of their profiles and can decide whether to share characteristics such as age, gender and ethnicity. The download from the forum that the researchers were provided with by HealthUnlocked associated each user with a numerical ID from which it was not possible to recover original usernames. Where potentially identifying information was accidentally retained in the download, the researchers removed any cases that were quoted in their analyses. In addition, the use of corpus methods further reduces the chances that a forum user's identity may be recoverable, as the findings of corpus linguistic analyses often involve aggregate information about frequencies of uses of words, phrases, collocational pairs and so on. Because of the settings of the HealthUnlocked site, it is also not possible to use search engines to trace back to the original post any verbatim quotation included in presentations or publications. Given that this corpus was obtained from HealthUnlocked, it cannot be redistributed, meaning that only researchers who paid to access the same data with HealthUnlocked could easily reach past the examples and aggregate data that the CASS team are allowed to publish. Yet even where such access is paid for, the data from HealthUnlocked is pre-anonymised, as noted. While the probability that a user may be identified as a result of research on the forums run by HealthUnlocked is extremely small, it nonetheless needs to be considered. Here the topic of the forum is relevant. Pain is a highly sensitive and potentially distressing experience, but it is not strongly stigmatised. In addition, potentially stigmatising statements (e.g., regarding suicidal ideation) were avoided in the selection of any verbatim quotations as part of the dissemination of the research. Conversely, as with all projects discussed in this book, Collins and Semino (2024) aimed to share relevant findings with Pain Concern and other relevant organisations and individuals, in order to maximise the potential benefits of the study, such as fostering better understanding of the experience of people affected by pain and improving language-based diagnostic questionnaires.

When forum contributors are given the chance to opt in or out of having their data used for research purposes, as in the case of HealthUnlocked forums, a potential limitation of working with the data is that some contributions are missing. As a result, certain 'conversations' on the forum, where people respond to one another's messages, may be incomplete, which makes it difficult to fully take into account the context of a forum post. Moreover, researchers have no way of knowing how many people opted out of having their data included. The findings of research are therefore limited to the posts of people who gave permission for their data to be used, as opposed to every person who posted to the forum, and this needs to be noted accordingly in any subsequent analysis.

Another potential issue with this kind of pre-anonymised data is the lack of full access to user information. Researchers are presented with information about posters' age, sex, and the country where they lived, for example, on the basis of what they provided when they signed up for an account. In the case of the Pain Concern forum, this information was useful in comparing the language use of different demographic groups, although researchers had no way of ascertaining the accuracy of the data provided about the posters. Additionally, as the analysis progressed, it became clear that some posters had created multiple accounts on the forum, sometimes leaving the forum, deleting their account and then rejoining later on. Because the data was pre-anonymised, it was not possible to identify every case where this occurred, so some posters would have been treated as more than one person, introducing an element of inaccuracy into our analysis. Again, such issues should be noted when reporting corpus findings.

To conclude on a practical note, as indicated, the contractual arrangement that facilitated the handling of ethical issues with regard to the Pain Concern forum required the payment of a fee to HealthUnlocked. Such data is therefore not easily accessible to all researchers, because access involves payment. It is therefore necessary to consider whether such payment is an allowable expense for research-funding applications and if it can be accommodated in the budget, as was the case for the grant that supported the project outlined in this section.

Overall, however, where funding is available, obtaining pre-anonymised forum data from contributors who had consented to their posts being used for research purposes makes it relatively easy to reconcile ethical considerations with the collection of large quantities of user-generated online data. With that said, it should be noted that this is not necessarily cheap. For the work undertaken by the team on two forums, a total of £17,000 was paid for access to forum data. While a good option for data access, the cost of such access probably precludes it as an option for many researchers.

4.3 Ethical Considerations When Working across Contexts and with Partners: Research on Public Discourses of Dementia

The work described previously provides, by way of a case study, insight into the kinds of ethical considerations that typically attend to a study of online health-related support groups. Such ethical considerations have, as we have seen, posed particular challenges for researchers using corpus linguistic techniques who, as part of their deliberations, are required to make judgments regarding, for example, the degree to which such contexts represent public or private settings. However, corpus research on health communication of course addresses a wide range of contexts and genres, including but also going beyond online support groups (see Brookes et al., 2022). As a way of addressing some of the various ethical considerations linked to such contexts and genres, as well as to cases of research programmes that involve

4.3 Ethical Considerations across Contexts with Partners   61

the participation of community and industry partners as research co-designers, we now consider the ethics underpinning the 'Public Discourses of Dementia' project.

4.3.1   Public Discourses of Dementia

The Public Discourses of Dementia project is a research programme which aims to identify and challenge stigma around dementia through analysis of the linguistic and visual and representations of dementia, and people diagnosed with dementia, across a wide range of contexts of public communication. The contexts under examination include, among others, newspaper articles, social media texts (i.e., tweets/posts on Twitter/X), campaigns produced by charities, and interactions in online support groups. Importantly, the researchers involved in the project have also worked closely with different partner groups, including people with a dementia diagnosis, dementia charities, healthcare professionals, and representatives from the media. This partner engagement began with the design of the project, which took place in conjunction with the researchers and partners, and has continued throughout the research programme. Further work is planned that will allow this collaborative approach to continue beyond the current project. The goal of this partnership is the co-production of sets of guidelines intended to support public communicators in writing about (and otherwise representing) dementia, and people diagnosed with it, in ways that can help to reduce the stigma surrounding the syndrome while promoting genuine awareness of it.

In collaboration with these project partners the academic research team was able to determine the contexts to be studied as part of the research. As discussed earlier in the chapter, some of these contexts, as sites of public communication, posed minimal ethical issues. For example, newspaper articles and public health campaigns produced by dementia charities, as texts that are freely available and designed for public consumption, did not require informed consent to be obtained from the producers of such texts or copyright holders prior to collection for analysis. However, redistributing such data would be a different matter and might require permissions to be sought, as would sharing screenshots of copyright-protected websites or copyright-protected images featured in such texts.

On the other hand, online support groups and social media texts required greater ethical consideration. Regarding the collection of texts from online support groups, the research was, much like the project examining language around pain described previously, based on data supplied by HealthUnlocked, which, as noted, was covered by blanket consent. For the collection of data from Twitter/X, approval needed to be sought from the institutional review board of the researchers' university and an application also had to be made to the Twitter/X API in order to enable programmatic access to posts on the site. Posts were then only collected from accounts that made their contributions publicly viewable (i.e., which did not require an account to access). In the case of both the HealthUnlocked data and the Twitter/X data, it was decided to remove identifying information from the corpus output (e.g., in concordance lines and extracts), to avoid supporting the easy identification of site users by readers of the academic publications in question. Our advice to researchers would be that while the underlying corpus data should remain inviolate, data presented from the corpus may, with issues of ethics in mind, be edited in a way which still allows the point illustrated to be made but does not allow for potentially sensitive information, irrelevant to that point, to be revealed. Where such editing of corpus data happens, the nature and motivation for it should be noted.

4.3.2 The Ethics of Co-design

Funding agencies and charitable organisations (in the United Kingdom, among other places) have increasingly required academic teams to clearly demonstrate how individuals with direct experience related to the research topic have been, or will be, actively engaged throughout the research process (Manafò et al., 2018). This involvement may cover various stages, from initial proposal development to more extensive roles in data collection, analysis and the dissemination of findings (Grand et al., 2015). In the context of health-related research, this practice is commonly known as Patient and Public Involvement (PPI). In recent years, as well as being involved in research in the aforementioned ways, it has also become more frequent for these individuals to play essential roles also in the design of research, including being part of academic teams applying for research funding (Swarbrick et al., 2019).

While such engagement can bring substantial benefits to the research process (Pizzo et al., 2015), and indeed to researchers themselves (Biggane et al., 2019), it does not come without challenges, including those of an ethical nature. Among other things, it is incumbent upon researchers to ensure the following: '(1) People with lived experience should feel enabled, not disabled, to take part; (2) Support and facilitation should be provided to meet the needs and abilities of the individual, not the condition; and (3) The relationship between academic researchers and those with lived experience should be based on a collaborative and reciprocal partnership' (Swarbrick et al., 2019: 3166). The benefits of PPI can be maximised, for the research, the researchers and partners (including people with 'lived experience') when such involvement begins early in the research cycle (Varkonyi-Sepp et al., 2017). In the Public Discourses of Dementia project, the researchers were keen to involve partners in the research as soon as possible, beginning, as noted, with ideation and research design.

4.3 Ethical Considerations across Contexts with Partners 63

The researchers on this project therefore had to start by clarifying what was meant by 'co-design'. They also had to set out which partners would be involved and how. Making these decisions early required initiating partner involvement early. It also, crucially, was important for being able to communicate openly with partners about the nature of what would be required of them. A key part of this communication related to ensuring that their needs and desires regarding their project involvement were both understood and met. Moreover, such decisions were important to settle on early, of course, for the purposes of applying for ethical approval through the institutional ethics review board. The process of making such decisions, and broadly mapping out the nature of partner involvement, was supported by consulting the work of others who have undertaken such work previously, to understand and potentially draw inspiration from how they undertook such engagement in an ethical way (see also Sendra, 2024).

At this point, it was important to consider the particular needs of the partner groups that were to be involved in the work, especially for the individuals with a diagnosis of dementia. Rather than applying a generic approach to PPI, the project team was helpfully able to draw on a framework designed for, and on the basis of, engagement with people with dementia. In particular, they drew upon elements of Swarbrick and co-authors' (2019) CO-researcher INvolvement and Engagement in Dementia (COINED) model. This model, which itself was co-designed with people with lived experience of dementia, sets out principles which should underpin the ways in which academics and partners (jointly termed 'co-researchers' within this model) collaborate for the purposes of designing and piloting materials, collecting data, understanding the findings, sharing the findings, translating findings into practice, evaluating the impacts of the research, and planning and undertaking future work. Furthermore, and importantly, the model is underpinned by ongoing consultation with co-researchers with lived experience. In the case of the Public Discourses of Dementia project, such ongoing consultation takes place through regular contact with a project advisory board comprising all key partner representatives. Where applicable, project funds are made available to board members to cover, for example, any reasonable travel and accommodation costs they might incur in travelling to meet in-person with other project team members. Project funds are also made available to enable ongoing training and support for all co-researchers involved in the research.

Partner engagement in the Public Discourses of Dementia project is something that has occurred throughout the life cycle of the research programme, then, and is planned to continue beyond the end of the project too. As noted, partners actively contributed to the design of the project, including determining the shape of the planned impact programme (i.e., the co-development of communication guidelines). This consultation also helped determine which contexts of public communication would be researched, ensuring that the findings, and resultant guidelines on which these were based, would represent key communicative contexts in terms of the formats that partners engaged with and which might be said to have a significant influence on shaping public attitudes towards dementia. In this way, the development of the advisory board was an iterative process, with partner ambassadors being invited on the recommendations of people with lived experience of dementia (e.g., in particular charities and advocacy groups), as well as in order to reflect the kinds of data to be studied (e.g., with the involvement of a journalist working with the BBC and another with a local newspaper).

In a practical sense, identifying and reaching out to partners may represent a challenge for the academic research team. As noted, some of the partners were approached on the recommendation of other advisory board members. In some of these cases, the partner representatives in question had offered to act as a point of contact and to facilitate initial engagement, which was arguably likely to be more effective than the academic research team simply getting in contact 'out of the blue'. In other cases, the academic research team were able to make contact on the basis of longer-term relationships with the partners in question, developed in many cases over many years and on the basis of meetings at events such as conferences and through participation in (dementia-themed) research groups. A particular challenge that has been raised in relation to research involving people with a dementia diagnosis concerns ensuring that the individuals in question have the appropriate capacity for consent (Cacchione, 2011). In this case, care was taken to approach people with lived experience of dementia through existing networks and infrastructure through which such individuals had already regularly participated in research, and indeed who had continued to participate in other research projects right up to and during the Public Discourses of Dementia programme.

The approach taken to engagement and co-design with the project partners in this programme of work was thus intended to ensure that the work was carried out in accordance with the Belmont Principles described at the beginning of this chapter. The project team respected the autonomy of the partners but was also mindful that some of the partners may have reduced autonomy (e.g., regarding issues surrounding capacity for consent in people with a diagnosis of dementia) and took special steps in this case, including by drawing on existing infrastructure at the university to make sure that the research process did not risk becoming exploitative of such individuals. This is also connected to the issue of beneficence – which, as noted, involves avoiding harm to people and maximising their well-being. In fact, this issue is at the very heart of the Public Discourses of Dementia project, which through linguistic analysis and the provision of evidence-based support for public communicators has sought to reduce the harmful stigma that surrounds dementia in public life, and to diversify the discourse and help facilitate more person-centred, life-affirming discourses in the process. Finally, the project design was also underpinned at all of its stages by the principle of justice. This, as mentioned, involves treating people equitably and making sure that the research benefits those most in need or most entitled to benefit. As the process of research co-design importantly involved people with a dementia diagnosis, the research team was able to design the project in a way that meant its aims and benefits were, as noted, responsive to the needs and perspectives of those living with dementia. Moreover, by continuing this engagement throughout the course of the project (and, importantly, beyond it), the team was able to ensure that such needs and perspectives also shaped how the project was carried out, while also confirming that the 'impact' activities undertaken at the conclusion of the academic research reached those most in need.

4.4 Conclusion

This chapter has, we hope, underscored the importance of ethical considerations in (corpus) linguistic research on healthcare communication. Ethical considerations are not merely procedural requirements but are fundamental to the integrity and societal value of research. The two case studies discussed in this chapter – the corpus-based study of an online pain forum and the Public Discourses of Dementia project – exemplify, among other things, the practical application of these ethical principles. They illustrate how ethical challenges can be navigated through, for example, careful planning, obtaining informed consent, ensuring anonymity and involving partners in the research process. These studies also emphasise the significance of patient and public involvement in enhancing the relevance and impact of research. Indeed, the importance and benefit of involving partners in the research design process cannot be overstated. Ethics in the social sciences often focuses on not doing harm. However, as we note in this chapter, it is also crucial to weigh this against the potential benefits of carrying out the research. Analysts need to ensure that their research findings can reach those who can benefit from them most, a topic we discuss in Chapter 12, which considers dissemination and impact.

Due to the larger scale necessitated by a corpus analysis, ethical considerations can appear especially daunting, particularly when collecting data related to sensitive health topics. By considering different types of linguistic data, ranging from material in the public domain to highly sensitive private communication, this chapter has also highlighted the contextual sensitivity that is required of such ethical scrutiny. While there is no one-size-fits-all solution to ethics, we hope that the case studies outlined in this chapter have helped provide some ideas about best practices while also pointing readers towards existing ethics guidelines that can be consulted. As an example, the aforementioned Belmont Principles can provide a useful framework for such reflexive ethical decision-making in research.

References

Beauchamp, T. L. and Childress, J. F. (2001). *Principles of Biomedical Ethics*. Oxford University Press.

Biggane, A. M., Olsen, M. and Williamson, P. R. (2019). PPI in Research: A Reflection from Early Stage Researchers. *Research Involvement and Engagement*, 5(35). https://doi.org/10.1186/s40900-019-0170-2.

British Association for Applied Linguistics (BAAL). (2021). *Recommendations on Good Practice in Applied Linguistics*. www.baal.org.uk/wp-content/uploads/2021/03/BAAL-Good-Practice-Guidelines-2021.pdf.

Brookes, G., Atkins, S. and Harvey, K. (2022). Corpus Linguistics and Health Communication: Using Corpora to Examine the Representation of Health and Illness. In A. O'Keeffe and M. McCarthy (eds.), *The Routledge Handbook of Corpus Linguistics*, 2nd ed. (pp. 615–28). Routledge.

Cacchione, P. Z. (2011). People with Dementia: Capacity to Consent to Research Participation. *Clinical Nursing Research*, 20(3), 223–7. https://doi.org/10.1177/1054773811415810.

Collins, L. and Baker, P. (2023). *Language, Discourse and Anxiety*. Cambridge University Press.

Collins, L. and Semino, E. (2024). An Analysis of Female and Male Opening Posts on an Online Forum Dedicated to Pain. *Journal of Language and Health*, 2(2), 100024. https://doi.org/10.1016/j.laheal.2024.07.001.

Demjén, Z., Atkins, S. and Semino, E. (2023). *Researching Health Communication*. Routledge.

Eysenbach, G., Powell, J., Englesakis, M., Rizo, C. and Stern, A. (2004). Health Related Virtual Communities and Electronic Support Groups: Systematic Review of the Effects of Online Peer to Peer Interactions. *BMJ*, 328, 1166. https://doi.org/10.1136/bmj.328.7449.1166.

Franzke, A. S., Bechmann, A., Zimmer, M., Ess, C. M. and the Association of Internet Researchers (2020). *Internet Research: Ethical Guidelines 3.0*. https://aoir.org/reports/ethics3.pdf.

Graham, S. L. and Hardaker, C. (2017). (Im)politeness in Digital Communication. In J. Culpeper, M. Haugh and D. Z. Kádár (eds.), *The Palgrave Handbook of Linguistic (Im)politeness* (pp. 785–814). Palgrave Macmillan.

Grand, A., Davies, G., Holliman, R. and Adams, A. (2015). Mapping Public Engagement with Research in a UK University. *PLoS ONE*, 10(4), e0121874. https://doi.org/10.1371/journal.pone.0121874.

Hunt, D. and Brookes, G. (2020). *Corpus, Discourse and Mental Health*. Bloomsbury.

Manafò, E., Petermann, L., Vandall-Walker, V. and Mason-Lai, P. (2018). Patient and Public Engagement in Priority Setting: A Systematic Rapid Review of the Literature. *PLoS ONE*, 13(3), e0193579. https://doi.org/10.1371/journal.pone.0193579.

Mackenzie, J. (2017). Identifying Informational Norms in Mumsnet Talk: A Reflexive-Linguistic Approach to Internet Research Ethics. *Applied Linguistics Review*, *8*(2–3), 293–314. https://doi.org/10.1515/applirev-2016-1042.

Pizzo, E., Doyle, C., Matthews, R. and Barlow, J. (2015). Patient and Public Involvement: How Much Do We Spend and What Are the Benefits? *Health Expectations*, *18*, 1918–26. https://doi.org/10.1111/hex.12204.

Sendra, P. (2024). The Ethics of Co-design. *Journal of Urban Design*, *29*(1), 4–22. https://doi.org/10.1080/13574809.2023.2171856.

Smith-Merry, J., Goggin, G., Campbell, A., McKenzie, K., Ridout, B. and Baylosis, C. (2019). Social Connection and Online Engagement: Insights from Interviews with Users of a Mental Health Online Forum. *Journal of Medical Internet Research: Mental Health*, *21*(3), e11084. https://doi.org/10.2196/11084.

Suler, J. (2004). The Online Disinhibition Effect. *CyberPsychology & Behavior*, 7(3), 321–6.

Swarbrick, C. M., Doors, O., EDUCATE, Davis, K. and Keady, J. (2019). Visioning Change: Co-producing a Model of Involvement and Engagement in Research (Innovative Practice). *Dementia*, *8*(7–8), 3165–72. https://doi.org/10.1177/1471301216674559.

Varkonyi-Sepp, J., Cross, A. and Howarth, P. (2017). Setting Up and Initiating PPI as a Collaborative Process Benefits Research in Its Early Stages. *Health Psychology Update*, *26*(2), 10–17. https://doi.org/10.53841/bpshpu.2017.26.2.10.

Yip, J. W. C. (2020). Evaluating the Communication of Online Social Support: A Mixed-Methods Analysis of Structure and Content. *Health Communication*, *35* (10), 1210–18. https://doi.org/10.1080/10410236.2019.1623643.

5 Interaction

5.1 Introduction

Healthcare typically involves the coming together of different perspectives and interaction between, for example, the individual with a health concern and the practitioner with the expertise to provide treatment, or peer-to-peer discussions online. In healthcare contexts, language can be used in dialogue to perform various social actions that can be highly consequential for our well-being. In this chapter we focus specifically on interactions as sequences of turns, in which a contribution is contingent upon what has come before and, indeed, has implications for the relevance of what follows. This thereby demonstrates the 'sequential implicativeness' (Schegloff and Sacks, 1967) of what participants contribute to the discussion of health issues. Furthermore, we demonstrate how the correspondence between contributions is what fosters community, as participants develop a shared language around health topics.

As mentioned in Chapter 4, online forums have become a popular resource through which individuals seeking health information and support can connect with a community, typically characterised by members with lived experience who can offer advice on working towards self-management (Hunt and Harvey, 2015). They constitute a space in which participants seek interaction with people who have relatable experiences, and the relative anonymity of such spaces encourages a high level of candour, as participants can discuss the particulars of their health concerns without necessarily sharing details of their personal identities (Frost et al., 2014). The peer-led nature of online forums also facilitates patient perspectives that are largely 'unedited' (Kinloch and Jaworska, 2020), compared with how patient contributions are reformulated in institutional settings according to the biomedical structures of patient forms and consultations. Studying these open, more egalitarian interactions (Chen and Chiu, 2008) can thus provide insights into how patients interact with peers for various communicative purposes.

We review two case studies of online forum exchanges, demonstrating different ways of using corpus analysis to identify patterns of interaction. Historically, analysts have combined corpus approaches predicated on the frequency and distribution of linguistics features with micro-analyses of the organisation of talk at the turn-by-turn level, drawing on concepts from conversation analysis (CA) or similar qualitative approaches (see Meredith, 2019) to look at interactional aspects. Atkins (2019: 113) recounts how corpus methods enabled her to identify the 'linguistic fingerprint' of a collection of simulated consultations in the form of recurring phrasal units; CA procedures subsequently helped provide insight into how interactional projects, such as eliciting patient histories or navigating interactional difficulties, were achieved at the micro-level (i.e., over the course of conversational turns). We similarly demonstrate how corpus procedures, specifically keyness analysis, provided a point of entry for our researchers to investigate how 'warfare' vocabulary was used as a collaborative humour strategy in an online forum for cancer support. We then refer to an anxiety support forum to discuss an alternative approach in which we used corpus tools to assist us in computing patterns for communication in terms of functions, having manually annotated the data according to discourse structures.

5.2 Co-constructed Humour on a Forum for People with Cancer

In this section we show how a corpus-based study of metaphors in an online forum dedicated to cancer led to the identification of patterns of humorous uses of language that required a sequential analysis of interactions among forum contributors. We begin by explaining how this particular phenomenon was initially identified within the larger study on metaphors for cancer (Semino et al., 2018). We then discuss the analytical reorientation that was required in order to explore to this phenomenon and the insights that this reorientation achieved.

5.2.1 A Corpus-Based Study of Metaphors for Cancer: The Accidental Discovery of Humorous Metaphors

As part of a project entitled 'Metaphor in End-of-Life Care' (MELC), a team based at Lancaster University employed a combination of corpus tools to analyse the use of metaphors for the experiences of cancer and the end of life. The 1.5-million-word corpus consisted of interviews with and online forum posts by members of three relevant stakeholder groups: people with cancer, unpaid carers looking after a person with cancer and healthcare professionals (Semino et al., 2018). The project was inspired, in part, by long-standing controversies surrounding the conventional metaphor of having cancer as a battle (e.g., 'fighting cancer') and the suggestion that it was more appropriate to use different metaphors, such as 'cancer journey' (Cancer Institute of New South Wales, 2023), or no metaphors at all (Sontag, 1979).

The MELC team found that what they call 'Violence' and 'Journey' metaphors are the two most frequently used types of metaphors in the data (Semino et al., 2018: 84). They also provided textual evidence of potentially harmful consequences of Violence metaphors, as when a forum contributor who has been told that her cancer has become incurable says, 'I feel such a failure that I am not winning this battle.' Here the feeling of failure seems to be generated by the metaphorical scenario in which the patient presents herself as 'not winning', in contrast with a 'literal' reality in which the disease cannot be cured because of the limitations of available treatments. However, the analysis of 899 instances of Violence metaphors in the online patient section of the MELC corpus also revealed that some contributors to the forum use them in 'empowering' ways, as in 'my consultants recognised that I was a born fighter'. Indeed, Semino and colleagues (2017) show that both Violence and Journey metaphors can be used in empowering and disempowering ways. They therefore argue that the implications of specific uses of metaphor in terms of (dis) empowerment are more important, particularly with respect to patients' wellbeing, than the type of metaphor involved (e.g., Violence versus Journey).

The team also noticed early on the humorous overtones that some of the metaphors carried, alongside presenting the person with cancer in a highly agentive, empowered position in relation to the disease. In the following examples, the humorous element arises from a combination of the metaphorical use of 'kicking' in relation to the cancer and the use of the informal expression 'butt' and the niche term 'wahoola'.

> Your words though have given me a bit more of my fighting spirit back. I am ready to kick some cancer butt!
>
> Don't let the Demon get you down, spit it in it's eye and give it a swift kick up the wahoola.

The presence of humour in discussions of a serious illness such as cancer may be unexpected but should not be entirely surprising. Humour is not just a central part of how, as human beings, we perceive the world and communicate with one another. It has also long been associated with three main functions (Attardo, 1994) that are relevant to coping with adversity: disparaging someone/something else (in our case, a serious illness, the health system, etc.); releasing negative emotions (in our case, the stress and anxiety associated with being ill); and creating intimacy and social bonds with others (in our case, people on an online forum who share the same illness).

Focussing on humour was not initially part of the team's plan for analysis. Having noticed this phenomenon while familiarising themselves with the data, however, the researchers explored the methodological issue of how to pursue the investigation of humour more systematically in the data.

5.2.2 Humorous Metaphors: From Serendipity to Corpus-Based Analyses

Humour does not have predictable linguistic realisations and is therefore not a straightforward phenomenon to investigate via corpus methods (but see Macqueen et al., 2024). However, by following up the instances of humour that they had come across serendipitously, the MELC team identified a particular thread on the cancer online forum which was entirely dedicated to humour.

The thread is entitled 'For those with a warped sense of humour WARNING – no punches pulled here' (henceforth 'Warped'). Due to the sampling approach that had been taken to create the MELC datasets, only a section of Warped was included in the MELC sub-corpus of online forum posts by patients. However, to carry out a thorough analysis of cancer-related humour, the team returned to the original data source to consider the complete Warped thread. At the time of data collection in 2012, it contained 2,544 posts contributed by 68 unique participants over 13 months, for a total of 530,055 words. This made it one of the largest of the 30,000 threads on the online forum of the UK-based cancer charity from which the team collected their data. Contributors to Warped take a humorous approach to a variety of topics, such as the side effects of treatment, irritations in the workplace, needing to buy new clothes and so on.

To identify the distinctive linguistic characteristics of Warped among the other threads on the forum, a keyness analysis was carried out (Semino et al., 2018: 240ff.; see Chapter 1 for a brief introduction). This involved using Warped as the target corpus and a 1-million-word corpus of contributions to the forum that *exclude* Warped as a reference corpus. A log likelihood cut-off of 10.83 was adopted (indicating that if there was no difference between the types of language use in the two sub-corpora, there is only a 0.01 per cent chance that the item in question would be key). Semino and co-authors show how several of the key parts of speech and key semantic domains revealed by the comparison contain humorous uses of language, including metaphorical ones. Here we will focus on a particular pattern that emerged from the combination of two key items: a key part of speech and a key semantic domain.

The key part of speech category is 'Preceding noun of title' (with the tag NNB), which includes words such as *Mr*, *Mrs*, and *Prof*. In Warped, the terms are used in light-hearted personifications of cancer (e.g., *Mr Crab*) and in the humorous use of military titles as nicknames that some of the contributors use for one another, such as *Flight Lieutenant Tom* and *Captain Joe*.

The key semantic domain is 'Warfare, defence and the army; weapons' (with the tag G3). This includes words such as *war*, *armed* and *bombing*. Its presence among the key semantic domains in Warped was remarkable because, as we have mentioned, Violence metaphors, which frequently involve war-related vocabulary, are one of the two most-frequent types of metaphors in the whole corpus and the most frequent in the sub-corpus of online contributions by patients. Given that this vocabulary can be expected in threads across the forum, why should these terms be used significantly more often in Warped? An initial examination of concordance lines showed that, in most cases, lexical items included under the 'Warfare, defence and the army; weapons' semantic domain were used metaphorically, and humorously, in relation to joint activities that forum contributors engage in:

> Cancer is the reason we are all here, so let's all fight that as an army together, chaaaaaaaaaaaaarge.

However, a more systematic analysis of concordance lines for both key items proved problematic, as it was often difficult to understand what was being talked about. Consider the following extract about one of the contributor's hospital test results (and note that all names/usernames in the quotes included in this chapter are replacements of the original names/usernames, following Semino and co-authors' (2018) approach to anonymisation):

> It's got to be good results Valerie or they've made a mistake. Don't forget we have a formidable fighting force in our rescue team which now has two successful missions under their belts. Tell them if they get it wrong we will all travel in Pretzel's bin to put it right.

What are the *missions* that the *fighting force* in the *rescue team* has successfully carried out? And what is the *bin* that the writers and others are supposed to *travel in*? Clearly the contributors shared some common ground that the researchers did not have, and this required going beyond concordance lines and reading substantial chunks from the Warped thread to understand what contributors are doing when they use the kind of vocabulary that accounted for the keyness of the 'Warfare, defence and the army; weapons' semantic domain.

5.2.3 Co-created Metaphorical Humour on a Forum Thread

By reading contributions to Warped sequentially, the team observed the origin, development and eventual demise of (metaphorical) in-jokes. With this additional context, references to the *fighting force*, as in the previously quoted extract, began to make sense. The co-creation of humour over extended stretches of interaction has been previously studied in informal oral interactions (Dynel, 2009) but has not yet received much attention in online discussions of illness experiences. The size of the Warped dataset made such an analysis, of this scale, possible.

Approximately a month after the inception of Warped in July 2011, some contributors started describing each other humorously as army officers on the same *camp*, giving one another titles such as *commandant*, *brigadier*, and

5.2 Co-constructed Humour on a Cancer Forum 73

colonel. These descriptions are initially used in relation to different imaginary enterprises that contributors would engage in if they met in person. In this context, perceived success is jokingly rewarded by promotion up the army ranks:

> Well done Flight lieutennant Tom for finding your way all the way over here from blog land ... I am impressed ... I would promote you but a) i think you have reached top rank already and b) I can't think of other ranks ... and not sure what the top one is ... I think Brigadeer is my favourite ... what's yours commander?

As the thread develops, the idea of Warped contributors as members of an army is used as part of an instantiation of the conventional metaphor whereby being ill with cancer is a fight against the disease:

> Cancer is the reason we are all here, so let's all fight that as an army together, chaaaaaaaaaaaaarge.

In early 2012, however, a particular combination of posts triggered a new development of the (conventional) metaphor of people with cancer as fighters. A contributor referred to by Semino and colleagues (2018) as 'Pretzel' tells the story of her attempt to dispose of an old fire alarm that was emitting a continuous sound by placing it in a wheelie bin due for collection on that day. However, the bin collectors did not turn up, leaving Pretzel with ongoing embarrassment at the sound emanating from the bin. This inspires several contributors to imagine the reaction of Pretzel's neighbours, including a scenario in which someone fears that the sound comes from an explosive device and calls *the bomb squad*. While this scenario is being developed, another contributor (Suzysue) metaphorically describes a longer-than-expected hospital stay as being *still imprisoned* by *warders*. This inspires another contributor to combine the imaginary wheelie bin scenario with the metaphor of hospitalised patients as prisoners and to propose that the group should use Pretzel's bin with the beeping smoke alarm as a distraction to get Suzysue *evacuated* and *liberated*.

From this point on, Warped contributors take turns to produce increasingly bizarre versions of metaphorical scenarios in which they are an army conducting rescue missions to liberate cancer patients from hospitals by using, among other things, Pretzel's wheelie bin. This leads to the kind of humorous metaphorical narrative that had initially flummoxed the MELC team when encountered in concordance lines:

> We need a plan of this prison, we don't want to rescue the wrong person. If you can send this to Pretzel who must stop the bin men emptying her wheelie bin. Pretztel if you can wheel your wheelie bin around to the main entrance of the prison, this will cause the distraction with everyone being evacuated through other entrances.

> as there has to be one as official armourer for warped I will put some balls of wool in the armoury may come in useful for launching from the bin at those most deserving

Semino and colleagues (2018) discuss the characteristics and functions of these chains of descriptions of metaphorical rescue missions. From the perspective of metaphor use, they involve the collaborative creative extension of the conventional metaphor of having cancer as a battle and cancer patients as fighters. In the rescue mission scenarios, the patients fight the health system rather than the illness and do so via rather unorthodox means. From a humour perspective, contributors co-create and co-develop an in-joke that makes light of a stressful situation (hospital stays) and that strengthens the bonds of solidarity and complicity between them. This can make a difficult situation easier to bear. Moreover, as Semino and colleagues (2018: 255) put it:

> They effectively become each other's heroes, subverting the usual rhetoric around cancer (Sandaunet, 2008) where patients are ideally brave fighters alone against cancer. In this way, they not only live through adventures together within the scenario, but they also manage to resist a dominant cultural framing of the cancer experience in real life.

Two further studies of metaphorical in-jokes on Warped have employed Dynamic Systems Theory (Larsen-Freeman and Cameron, 2008) to explain the way in which these humorous metaphors emerge, are collaboratively developed and eventually decline (Semino and Demjén, 2017; Demjén, 2018). From this perspective, the interactions on the Warped thread 'can be seen as a self-organizing system which evolves over multiple time-scales as a result of complex interactions between internal and external forces' (Semino and Demjén, 2017: 186). Humorous metaphors such as those we have discussed are seen as emerging from the dynamic interaction between external factors, such as the conventional metaphors of having cancer as a battle, and internal factors, such as the nature of the Warped thread and previous posts by contributors (Gibbs and Cameron, 2008). The development of humorous metaphors over time involves patterns of both stability and variation. For example, Pretzel's story about the wheelie bin causes a perturbation in the system that results in a new metaphorical scenario, where rescue missions from hospitals involve the beeping wheelie bin. This scenario then becomes established as a pattern of stability in the system, until it eventually stops being used around July 2012 (six months after the first reference to the wheelie bin), as the community focuses on other patterns of shared humour.

5.3 Sequences of Communicative Purposes in an Online Anxiety Support Forum

Our second case study involves an online support forum for anxiety disorders, hosted by the digital platform HealthUnlocked, which we introduced in Chapter 4. Data collected from this Anxiety Support forum produced a corpus of 294,082 comments involving 17,770 different contributors between the

5.3 Sequences of Communicative Purposes in an Anxiety Forum

period 20 March 2012 and 14 September 2020. The structure of the exchanges that took place in the forum provided an opportunity to investigate how participants might set a conversational agenda with a post to initiate a discussion thread and how other members of the forum responded to develop the conversation. As reported in Collins and Baker (2023), there was great variability in how many responses a post initiating a discussion thread (what we call an Opening post) received, with 7.11 per cent of Opening posts receiving zero responses and 42.69 per cent of Opening posts receiving only one or two replies. Nevertheless, since a single discussion thread could contain up to 314 contributions, there was still ample opportunity to look at the interactional dynamics of messages in the forum – including why certain posts did not get many responses (see Collins and Baker, 2023: chapter 4).

5.3.1 Response Structure in Online Forums

While online forums function to host a potentially endless variety of conversation topics, there is a reasonably consistent structure across platforms that reflects their asynchronous, multiparty affordances (Morzy, 2013). Most online forums involve some degree of threading, visually indicating continuity between posts in the way that demonstrates their topical contiguity, even when a message is posted sometime after the post to which it responds. In light of this asynchronicity, respondents can use a range of features to maintain coherence when their messages are often not the next contribution to the discussion, chronologically speaking, such as lexical repetition and lexical substitution (Meredith, 2019: 247), or even explicitly targeting the recipient of their post through @-tagging.

In its naturally occurring form, the thread of forum posts is typically represented visually on the forum interface, providing a kind of flow diagram of the conversation. When these online interactions are encoded in plain text for the purposes of (corpus) analysis, these thread relations can be documented as metadata. HealthUnlocked provided the forum data to the researchers as a spreadsheet with metadata in columns alongside the message content. Table 5.1 shows a simplified version of the spreadsheet information and demonstrates how the structure of discussion threads across the forum is captured according to thread and message identifiers (Thread ID, Parent ID, Post ID). The examples shown in Table 5.1 represent the complete set of contributions to the discussion thread 1241, with each post given a unique numerical identifier (Post ID) and a timestamp indicating when it was posted.

Each post is also given a Parent ID, which corresponds with the Post ID of the message 'under' which the contribution was posted as a response; for example, the second row in Table 5.1 was posted as a direct reply to the Opening post (Post ID: 1241) and the third contribution was posted as a reply to the second message.

76　　5 Interaction

Table 5.1 *Forum post metadata for discussion thread 1241*

Thread ID	Parent ID	Post ID	Timestamp	User ID	Message content (excerpt)
None	None	1241	2016-11-08 10:22:56	#001	Title: Relentless Hi folks, im new to this page, i...
1241	1241	3289	2016-11-08 17:16:19	#002	It is so miserable it just is...
1241	3289	3394	2016-11-08 17:38:45	#001	Its the worst, i just feel so...
1241	3394	3415	2016-11-08 17:43:38	#002	I know exactly how you feel...
1241	3415	3443	2016-11-08 17:48:07	#001	I seen another comnent u posted...
1241	3443	3466	2016-11-08 17:50:41	#002	I am totally terrified of the jittery...
1241	3466	3471	2016-11-08 17:51:34	#001	I will do xx...
1241	3394	7904	2016-11-09 16:31:23	#003	I do that too! I keep my bedroom...
1241	7904	8456	2016-11-09 18:14:06	#001	Its awful to feel like this, its...
1241	8456	8484	2016-11-09 18:20:38	#003	I hope you can talk to your dr...
1241	8484	8533	2016-11-09 18:32:11	#001	Iv a lot of ailments and recently...
1241	8533	8548	2016-11-09 18:36:03	#003	If you have something that works...
1241	8548	8562	2016-11-09 18:37:48	#001	Me too, constant battle with my...

By referring to the User ID, we can see that the discussion involved three different contributors and that it was the original poster (#001) who returned to reply, first to participant #002 and then user #003.

While Table 5.1 presents the contributions chronologically, showing that the entire discussion thread took place between 10:22 a.m. on 8 November 2016 and 6:37 p.m. on 9 November 2016, Figure 5.1 demonstrates the response structure between the three contributors to the discussion thread. From this, we can see that user #003 responded not to the Opening post (Post ID: 1241) but rather to post 3394, which came from the initial exchange between users #001 and #002. While there is no direct interaction between users #002 and #003, it is important to remember that all posts are visible to those who visit the discussion thread (and may not post).

5.3 Sequences of Communicative Purposes in an Anxiety Forum 77

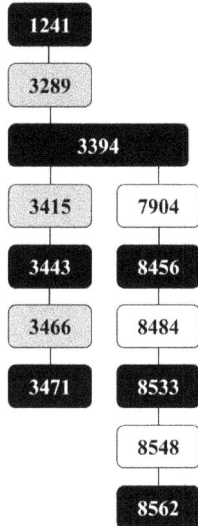

Figure 5.1 Response structure for discussion thread 1241.

5.3.2 Coding Discourse Units

With an understanding that online forums are characterised as providing information and emotional support (Yip, 2020), Collins and Baker referred to the framework developed by Biber and colleagues (2021) to capture the functional units of interactions. In other words, we can refer to 'discourse units' (DUs) to document how participants in the forum achieve communicative goals such as 'giving advice and instructions' or 'describing or explaining the past' in this digital, multi-party asynchronous mode.

The coding of discourse units is also described in Egbert and colleagues (2021: 725), wherein the authors provide their operational definition for a discourse unit as follows:

1. Coherent for its overarching communicative goal, which is both the primary objective of the DU and the task that the interlocutors are doing with language in the DU
2. Characterised by one or more communicative purposes, where a communicative purpose is a finite set of actions that serve to help accomplish the communicative goal of a DU
3. Recognisably self-contained: a DU has an identifiable beginning and end

Egbert and colleagues (2021) explain that the range of possibilities for communicative goals (which might be complaining about annoying co-workers or making plans for buying Christmas presents) is boundless and so not coded. However, they developed a taxonomy for nine types of *communicative purpose*, which are summarised in Table 5.2. In their application of this taxonomy to examine informal spoken conversations, the authors also found that imposing a length requirement optimised the coding between raters and so established the additional criterion:

4. A discourse unit has a minimum of five utterances or 100 words.

Similarly motivated by reaching optimal agreement between coders, Collins and Baker (2023) forewent a length requirement when coding discourse units in the Anxiety Support forum data, finding that the communicative purpose 'giving advice and instructions', for example, could be observed in a short forum contribution such as 'You should go see your GP'.

Table 5.2 *Biber et al.'s (2021) taxonomy for nine communicative purposes*

Label	Abbreviation	Summary
Situation-dependent commentary	sdc	This purpose occurs when speakers in a conversation are commenting on people or objects that are present, or events that are occurring in their shared situational context.
Joking around	jok	This includes conversation that is intended to be humorous, including both light-hearted and darker humour. It also includes good-humoured banter, teasing and flirting.
Engaging in conflict	con	This purpose includes disagreement of any type, including more light-hearted debate as well as more serious quarrelling.
Figuring things out	fto	This purpose encapsulates discussion aimed at exploring or considering options or plans, including discussion about how things work and what the best solution to a problem may be.
Sharing feelings and evaluations	fel	This includes discussion about feelings, evaluations, opinions and beliefs, including the airing of grievances and the sharing of personal perspectives.
Giving advice and instructions	adv	This occurs when one speaker offers directions, advice or suggestions to another speaker.
Describing or explaining the past	pas	This purpose includes narrative stories about true events from the past or other references to people or events from the past.
Describing or explaining the future	fut	This includes descriptions or speculations about future events and intentions, including those that are planned and those that are more hypothetical.
Describing or explaining (time-neutral)	des	Descriptions or explanations about facts, information, people or events where time (past or future) is either irrelevant or unspecified.

5.3 Sequences of Communicative Purposes in an Anxiety Forum 79

The nine communicative purposes, as described in Biber and colleagues (2021: 25), are presented in Table 5.2.

Through their application of the coding framework, Biber and colleagues (2021) recognised that an individual DU can serve multiple communicative purposes and so implemented the tags according to a 0–3 quantitative scale in which 0 = purpose not present (not recorded), 1 = minor purpose, 2 = major purpose and 3 = dominant purpose. To demonstrate this, we have produced the full message of the Opening post of discussion thread 1241 in Table 5.3, showing how the post can be divided into two DUs and how each DU was coded according to its dominant and additional functions. This coding reflects our reading of the post as beginning with situation-dependent commentary, through references to *this page* and the forum more generally, before the contributor expresses the difficult feelings they are experiencing (the communicative purpose fel) while also offering a description of their experiences of anxiety (the communicative purpose des).

Collins and Baker (2023) report the occurrence of each communicative purpose across a randomised sample of one discussion thread from each calendar month of the data, which amounted to 103 discussion threads, comprising 822 individual posts. They found that the most common communicative purpose observed was the expression of opinions and personal perspectives (fel), followed by explanations (des) and advice-giving (adv), with minimal occurrences of conflict communication (con) and joking (jok) in the forum interactions.

5.3.3 Sequences of Discourse Units

The coding of discourse units enabled Collins and Baker (2023) to consider not only how communicative purposes were combined in one discourse unit but

Table 5.3 *Discourse unit coding for an Opening forum post (Post ID: 1241)*

	Communicative purpose		
Message content	3	2	1
Title: Relentless Hi folks, im new to this page, i just needed somewhere to go to get my anxiety dwn into words,	sdc	–	–
i feel im at my wits end for months now iv lived with my anxiety from the minute i open my eyes until i fall asleep then im anxious in my dreams its never ending, i constantly feel sick my heart beats so hard i can hear it, iv no patience im extremely emotional i get so wound up i become breathless, i constantly think bad is going to happen, how do i cope with this, its takin over my life and im at a loss as to wot to do	fel	des	–

also how discourse units were combined within a single forum post. For example, the message in Table 5.3 carries both the communicative purpose of discussing something in the shared situational context of the visitors to the forum (i.e., the forum itself) and conveying their personal perspective. As was the case with Biber and colleagues (2021), Collins and Baker found that it was common for messages to serve multiple communicative purposes; for example, the pas code was used alongside explanations or advice-giving to provide a context drawn from lived experience. The researchers also discuss resultant communicative purposes in replies according to Opening posts that are characterised according to a particular communicative purpose (i.e., discussion threads initiated by Sharing feelings and opinions (fel)). However, they report that even when the communicative purpose of an Opening post appears to invite advice or explanations (such as an Opening post characterised in terms of 'figuring things out'), respondents seemed to prefer to present their recommendations indirectly, as personal perspectives (i.e., fel).

Here, we discuss the contributions to discussion thread 1241 to consider the extent to which the communicative purpose of the posts is informed by the purposes and structure of preceding messages. Ultimately, the aim of this application of the framework for coding discourse units is to focus on the sequencing of discussion threads to consider the interactional dynamics of how different communicative purposes are realised in the forum and how members create a dialogue that pursues particular communicative goals.

Table 5.4 demonstrates the communicative purpose codes applied to the discourse units we identified in comments appearing as part of discussion thread 1241. The shaded rows indicate the messages posted by the author of the Opening post. From this, we can see that there are 22 DUs, that 6 of the 13 posts included more than 1 DU and that the number of DUs in a post ranged from 1 to 4. Five of the nine communicative purposes are represented in this discussion and 13 (59.09 per cent) of the DUs were coded as having more than one communicative purpose.

If we refer back to the Opening post, as shown in full in Table 5.3, there is an apparent prompt for advice in the contributor's question, 'How do I cope with this?', and they assert that they are 'at a loss as to wot to do'. Collins and Baker (2023) report that many participants seem to post to the forum when they have exhausted their options or coping strategies and seek recommendations from other members. It is curious, then, to see that in response to this Opening post, User #002 does offer a contribution that functions as advice (which is for User #001 to *check out* User #002's profile page for a list of recommended responses that have helped them), but here User #002's dominant communicative purpose is to express their own personal perspective (fel), including the empathic statement *I feel your pain*. Thus, User #002 has foregrounded this display of empathy and emotional support over giving advice, which was directly requested.

5.3 Sequences of Communicative Purposes in an Anxiety Forum   81

Table 5.4 *Coding for communicative purposes of discourse units in the thread 1241*

Post ID/DU	Message content (excerpt)	Communicative purpose 3	2	1
1241/1	Title: Relentless//Hi folks, im new to this page,…	sdc	–	–
1241/2	i feel im at my wits end for months now…	fel	des	–
3289/1	It is so miserable it just is…	fel	adv	–
3394/1	Its the worst, i just feel so trapped,…	fel	–	–
3394/2	i dont leave the house, im even scared to close my blinds…	des	fel	–
3415/1	I know exactly how you feel…	fel	des	–
3415/2	I don't think the problem is in our head…	des	–	–
3415/3	But, just remind yourself, you are not alone…	adv	fut	–
3443/1	I seen another comnent u posted about medication,…	sdc	–	–
3443/2	my sister has some anxiety but not at my level…	des	adv	–
3443/3	im honestly thinkin of ringin my doc in the mornin…	fut	–	–
3443/4	good luck in ur search for help, its an awful way to live xx	fel	–	–
3466/1	I am totally terrified of the jittery feeling…	fel	fut	–
3466/2	Keep me updated if you do try it and if it is helpful!! :)	adv	–	fut
3471/1	I will do xx	fut	–	–
7904/1	I do that too! I keep my bedroom curtains open…	des	–	fel
8456/1	Its awful to feel like this, its dictating my life,…	fel	des	–
8484/1	I hope you can talk to your dr.	fel	–	–
8484/2	I do leave the house to work normally because I have…	des	–	fel
8533/1	Iv a lot of ailments and recently came off 25 tablets a day…	des	–	–
8548/1	If you have something that works I say take it if you can!…	des	adv	–
8562/1	Me too, constant battle with my thoughts and fear, its so hard…	des	fel	–

User #001 and User #002 then continue to trade messages (Post IDs 3394, 3415) that are characterised by the expression of feelings (fel) about the difficulties of their respective anxiety experiences, which is combined with explanations (des) as to how the effects of anxiety manifest in their day-to-day activities and how they try to cope. User #003 also demonstrates this reciprocal sharing of personal perspectives, picking up on the description from User #001 in post 3394 and going on to explain their own ways of coping in posts 7904, 8404 and 8548. We are reminded of the significance of finding a community of individuals who can appreciate such struggles in an exchange where User #002 states, 'No one understands what you're going through unless they have been through it too' (Post ID: 3289). Other users respond by reassuring 'it's all in your head' (Post ID: 3415) and User #001 similarly asserts that 'its so hard to get ppl to understand who havnt experienced it' (Post ID: 8562).

While there appears to be an impetus to demonstrate mutuality, as shown in User #003's contribution, 'I do that too!', there is also the recognition that anxiety experiences and coping strategies may differ for each individual: 'If you have something that works I say take it if you can!' Nevertheless, having established mutuality, the conversation between User #001 and User #002 appears to shift towards advice-giving (adv) and thinking ahead to the next steps (fut), as observed in the progression of post 3415 and post 3466. Thus, it would appear that both User #002 and User #003 work to establish reciprocity and a shared understanding of the difficult feelings associated with anxiety before proffering advice and looking ahead to what User #001, in particular, will do next. Establishing this understanding arguably puts them in a more legitimate position to offer advice and equally, for their recommendations to be taken on board by the original poster.

In this brief examination of a short sequence of posts within a discussion thread, we have shown how the coding of communicative purposes has helped document how social actions such as establishing mutuality, showing empathy, offering advice and planning for the future are achieved over the course of an interaction. With the appropriate annotation for these distinct code categories in place, analysts can use corpus tools to investigate the frequency, distribution, combination and sequence of such communicative purposes to investigate patterns in the dynamics of how users attend both to those communicative purposes elicited by other members, such as a request for advice, and what they perceive to be the communicative functions of platforms such as online support forums.

5.4 Conclusion

We have shown in this chapter how approaches to investigating interactions around health topics can variously combine corpus approaches and qualitative analysis. In the first case study, we showed that engagement with the extended co-text helped shed light on the significance of key features (titular nouns and warfare vocabulary) to the collaborative humour developed among an online community dealing with the challenges associated with cancer. In the second case study, the manual coding of discourse units highlighted how users prioritise different communicative purposes (such as expressing empathy), even if other communicative functions appeared to be elicited in the original post. Digital platforms, such as online forums, provide an archive of interactions, which allows participants to familiarise themselves with the conventions of the community space. Researchers can similarly mine this archive using corpus tools to systematically examine the forms and functions through which members negotiate community norms via interaction and thereby foster the types of exchange that have proven so valuable to individuals coping with illness.

References

Atkins, S. (2019). Assessing Health Professionals' Communication through Role-Play: An Interactional Analysis of Simulated versus Actual General Practice Consultations. *Discourse Studies*, *21*(2), 109–34. https://doi.org/10.1177/1461445618802659.

Attardo, S. (1994). *Linguistic Theories of Humor*. Mouton de Gruyter.

Biber, D., Egbert, J., Keller, D. and Wizner, S. (2021). Towards a Taxonomy of Conversational Discourse Types: An Empirical Corpus-Based Analysis. *Journal of Pragmatics*, *171*, 20–35. https://doi.org/10.1016/j.pragma.2020.09.018.

Cancer Institute of New South Wales. (2023). *Writing about Cancer Guidelines*. https://bit.ly/2Z93O5G. Accessed 19 December 2024.

Chen, G. and Chiu, M. M. (2008). Online Discussion Processes: Effects of Earlier Messages' Evaluations, Knowledge Content, Social Cues and Personal Information on Later Messages. *Computers & Education*, *50*(3), 678–92. https://doi.org/10.1016/j.compedu.2006.07.007.

Collins, L. C. and Baker, P. (2023). *Language, Discourse and Anxiety*. Cambridge University Press.

Demjén, Z. (2018). Complexity Theory and Conversational Humour: Tracing the Birth and Decline of a Running Joke in an Online Cancer Support Community. *Journal of Pragmatics*, *133*, 93–104. https://doi.org/10.1016/j.pragma.2018.06.001.

Dynel, M. (2009). Beyond a Joke: Types of Conversational Humour. *Language and Linguistics Compass*, *3*(5), 1284–99. https://doi.org/10.1111/j.1749-818X.2009.00152.x.

Egbert, J., Wizner, S., Keller, D., Biber, D., McEnery, T. and Baker, P. (2021). Identifying and Describing Functional Discourse Units in the BNC Spoken 2014. *Text & Talk*, *41*(5–6), 715–37. https://doi.org/10.1515/text-2020-0053.

Frost, J., Vermeulen, I. E. and Beekers, N. (2014). Anonymity versus Privacy: Selective Information Sharing in Online Cancer Communities. *Journal of Medical Internet Research*, *16*(5), e126. https://doi.org/10.2196/jmir.2684.

Gibbs, R. W. and Cameron, L. (2008). The Social-Cognitive Dynamics of Metaphor Performance. *Cognitive Systems Research*, *9*(1–2), 64–75. https://doi.org/10.1016/j.cogsys.2007.06.008.

Hunt, D. and Harvey, K. (2015). Health Communication and Corpus Linguistics: Using Corpus Tools to Analyse Eating Disorder Discourse Online. In P. Baker and T. McEnery (eds.), *Corpora and Discourse Studies: Integrating Discourse and Corpora* (pp. 134–54). Palgrave Macmillan.

Kinloch, K. and Jaworska, S. (2020). Using a Comparative Corpus-Assisted Approach to Study Health and Illness Discourses across Domains: The Case of Postnatal Depression (PND) in Lay, Medical and Media Texts. In Z. Demjén (ed.), *Applying Linguistics in Illness and Healthcare Contexts* (pp. 73–98). Bloomsbury.

Larsen-Freeman, D. and Cameron, L. (2008). *Complex Systems and Applied Linguistics*. Oxford University Press.

Macqueen, S., Collins, L., Brookes, G., Demjén, Z., Semino, E. and Slade, D. (2024). Laughter in Hospital Emergency Departments. *Discourse Studies*, *26*(3), 358–80. https://doi.org/10.1177/14614456231194845.

Meredith, J. (2019). Conversation Analysis and Online Interaction. *Research on Language and Social Interaction*, *52*(3), 241–56. https://doi.org/10.1080/08351813.2019.1631040.

Morzy, M. (2013). Evolution of Online Forum Communities. In T. Özyer, J. Rokne, G. Wagner and A. Reuser (eds.), *The Influence of Technology on Social Network Analysis and Mining. Lecture Notes in Social Networks*, vol 6. (pp. 615–30). Springer. https://doi.org/10.1007/978-3-7091-1346-2_27.

Sandaunet A. G. (2008). A Space for Suffering? Communicating Breast Cancer in an Online Self-Help Context. *Qualitative Health Research*, *18*(12), 1631–41. https://doi.org/10.1177/1049732308327076.

Schegloff, E. and Sacks, H. (1967). Opening Up Closings. *Semiotica*, *8*(4), 289–327. https://doi.org/10.1515/semi.1973.8.4.289.

Semino, E. and Demjén, Z. (2017). The Cancer Card: Metaphor, Intimacy and Humour in Online Interactions about the Experience of Cancer. In B. Hampe (ed.), *Metaphor: Embodied Cognition & Discourse* (pp. 181–99). Cambridge University Press.

Semino, E., Demjén, Z., Demmen, J., Koller, V., Payne, S., Hardie, H. and Rayson, P. (2017). The Online Use of 'Violence' and 'Journey' Metaphors by Cancer Patients, as Compared with Health Professionals: A Mixed Methods Study. *BMJ Supportive and Palliative Care*, *7*(1), 60–6. http://dx.doi.org/10.1136/bmjspcare-2014-000785.

Semino, E., Demjén, Z., Hardie, A., Payne, S. and Rayson, P. (2018). *Metaphor, Cancer and the End of Life: A Corpus-Based Study*. Routledge. https://doi.org/10.4324/9781315629834.

Sontag, S. (1979). *Illness as Metaphor*. Allen Lane.

Yip, J. W. C. (2020). Evaluating the Communication of Online Social Support: A Mixed-Methods Analysis of Structure and Content. *Health Communication*, *35*(10), 1210–18. https://doi.org/10.1080/10410236.2019.1623643.

6 Language Use and Identity

6.1 Introduction

The topic of identity has long been of interest to researchers in linguistics, including in the context of health communication. The term *identity* emerged in social science literature during the 1950s, with studies on the topic tending to fall into one of two broad categories; the first involves viewing identity as 'intrapsychic' (i.e., as an internal and fixed quality that reflects 'who we really are'), while the second views identity as a socially constructed role that is acquired or even imposed (Gleason, 1983). Between these categories is the notion of 'ego identity' (Habermas, 1975), which represents a socialised sense of individuality (Baker, 2010: 10). Research in the social sciences had tended to view identity in the second sense identified by Gleason (1983). Indeed, Preece (2016: 3) describes a shift in (applied) linguistic research 'from viewing identity as a set of fixed characteristics that are learned or biologically based to seeing identity as a social construct'.

Language use, or 'discourse', is one of the ways in which identity can be socially constructed. As Burr (2004: 106) puts it, identities are 'constructed out of the discourses culturally available to us, and which we draw upon in our communications with other people'. Importantly, this process is never static or 'complete' but, rather, is active, ongoing and dynamic (Benwell and Stokoe, 2006: 4). For linguists working in fields such as discourse analysis and sociolinguistics, an important consideration is how we might go about actually identifying the kinds of language use or discourses that people use to construct identities. As we will see in Chapter 10, we can approach the construction of identity from a perspective of representation, for example, by studying the language used to represent particular social actors or groups. Another way we can study identity, though, is to examine the language used by a given social actor or group of interest, to get a sense of how their identities are reflected in, and indeed constructed through, the language they use. This latter perspective is the focus of this chapter.

Corpus studies of language and identity often use annotation as a way of marking up the language in the corpus according to the relevant demographic characteristics of the language users represented within it (Baker, 2010). Annotation at the text level is likely to indicate the genre or mode of the texts contained within the corpus. Annotation at the linguistic level, meanwhile, usually indicates a word's grammatical class or the semantic field to which it belongs (Leech, 1997). In this chapter we focus on the use of annotation to study identity: the annotation of a corpus using demographic metadata relating to the characteristics of the language users represented within it, for instance relating to their age or sex identity (Baker, 2010). For example, when investigating sex, language users might be grouped into categories such as male, female, non-binary, and so forth (Baker, 2014; Baker and Brookes, 2021). Meanwhile, for age the groupings may reflect different age groups such as adolescents, people in their twenties, people in their thirties and so on. The annotations reflecting these categories can be used to divide the corpus into a series of sub-corpora which can then form the basis of an analysis, allowing us to focus on particular groups (e.g., men) or cross-sections of groups (e.g., men in their thirties), or to compare patterns across different groups (e.g., to compare people in their thirties against people in their forties). Thus, annotation has become particularly important to corpus linguistics because it can facilitate more complex and sophisticated analyses.

However, not all researchers will need to, or even *want* to, use annotation in their research. For many studies, it is possible to carry out analyses, including of identity, without the help of annotation. Meanwhile, some researchers regard annotation rather negatively, and it has been argued (e.g., by Sinclair, 1992) that annotation imposes upon the theoretical purity of the corpus and that the particular tags have the potential to be applied inconsistently or inaccurately. Once a suitable taxonomy has been established, we can employ corpus tools to automatically apply tags according to our instructions and can supplement this automated process by manually checking and correcting erroneous tags assigned to a corpus by a computational tagger. However, we should also bear in mind that the larger the corpus we are dealing with, the more laborious and less practical this process of manual checking becomes. Yet, even if we do want to perform annotation on our corpus data because we believe that it will support our analysis, it might not be possible for us to do so if we do not possess the information or metadata necessary to reliably tag the corpus in a way that would be relevant to our research. This obstacle is particularly relevant when using annotation to study identity, as the application of demographic tags depends on the annotator having access to reliable demographic metadata about the language users featured in the corpus. However, such information is not always available, especially when studying anonymous (particularly online) communicative contexts.

In this chapter we present two case studies which demonstrate how we might go about incorporating the consideration of language users' identities into a corpus analysis. First, we present an analysis of identity in a corpus of health communication data for which demographic metadata about the language users in the corpus *was* available. Second, we present an analysis of identity in a corpus containing texts belonging to a similar genre of health communication, but for which reliable demographic metadata was not available to the researchers (see Section 2.4 for background discussion relating to these studies). Taken together, the case studies presented over the coming pages respectively demonstrate, on the one hand, the affordances of demographic annotation for studying identity and, on the other hand, how as analysts we might work around a lack of such annotations in order to study identity in a corpus of health communication data.

6.2 Using Demographic Metadata

The first case study we present in this chapter, as noted, involves the use of demographic metadata annotation to study identity in a corpus of health communication data. Specifically, the study in question examines language use and sex identity in a corpus of patient evaluations of cancer care services in England (Baker and Brookes, 2022). It is worth first briefly discussing the notion of patient feedback and the context of the patients' evaluations. Since the 1980s, patient feedback exercises have been undertaken by an increasing number of healthcare providers across the globe in order to monitor the quality of the services they provide and stimulate improvements where these might be needed (Vingerhoets et al., 2001). While the reliability of patient feedback as an indicator of the technical quality of care can be debated (Coulter, 2006), it has nevertheless become a staple way of measuring and regulating healthcare standards (Graham and Woods, 2013) while also ensuring public involvement in the design and improvement of healthcare provision (Coulter, 2013).

6.2.1 *The Corpus and Its Context: Patient Feedback on Cancer Services in England*

Patient feedback can be obtained in a variety of ways, and the data analysed in this study was a specialised corpus of written feedback on cancer care services provided by patients responding to England's Cancer Patient Experience Survey (CPES). Responses were provided both through online and so-called pen-and-paper forms, with the latter subsequently being digitised to render them amenable to computational corpus analysis. The CPES form allows patients to provide both quantitative and qualitative feedback. The quantitative part of the form asks, 'Overall, how would you rate your care?', to which patients can respond by providing a score between 0 and 10, where a score of 0 indicates that they definitely would not recommend a service and a score of 10 indicates that they definitely would recommend it. Respondents could then describe their experiences and explain the score they gave by providing qualitative feedback across three free-text boxes preceded by the following questions: 'Was there anything particularly good about your NHS cancer care?'; 'Was there anything that could have been improved?'; and 'Any other comments?'. For the purposes of this study, all the comments each patient provided were combined to form a single 'text' (i.e., one text per piece of feedback).

The resulting corpus comprised 214,340 comments (14,403,694 words), relating to cancer services provided in England between 2015 and 2018. This data was made available to the researchers by NHS England's Insight and Feedback team in a spreadsheet format in which each comment was accompanied by details about each patient's care and certain socio-demographic characteristics. Some of these details were obtained by the organisation from patient records, while others were provided by the patients themselves, as requested on the feedback form. The researchers then used this metadata to annotate each comment with details about the patient who provided it. These included details relating to the patients' treatment, including the duration of treatment and the site on which they received it, as well as about their identity, including age, ethnicity, first language, sex, and sexuality. Here we focus on the analysis based on sex.

6.2.2 Analysis of Language and Sex Identity Based on Demographic Metadata

There were three options for patient sex in the CPES form: 'Male', 'Female' and 'Prefer not to say'. The vast majority of patients did respond to this question on the form, with approximately 54 per cent of the respondents identifying as female and approximately 46 per cent identifying as male. The researchers mounted the corpus on CQPweb (Hardie, 2012) and used the sex-related tags to divide the corpus into two sub-corpora: one containing comments provided by female patients and the other containing comments provided by male patients.

To compare the language used by these groups, the researchers then compared these sub-corpora against each other using the keywords technique (introduced in Chapter 1). Specifically, they generated two sets of keywords: one by using the male comments sub-corpus as the target and comparing it against the female comments sub-corpus as the reference, and the second by swapping these around and using the female comments sub-corpus as the target and the male comments sub-corpus as the reference. The resulting sets of keywords represent language use that was characteristic, respectively, of male and female patients' comments, when compared with each other. The following list shows the top-30 keywords for male patient comments, compared to female patients' comments (ranked by frequency (in brackets))[1]. These keywords were obtained using log likelihood (Dunning, 1993) with a log ratio cut-off (Hardie, 2014).

class (4,969), treatment (46,228), hospital (39,990), good (25,776), no (23,674), by (20,851), (18,719), GP (15,544), first (13,534), NHS (12,360), yes (7,509), months (6,853), blood (6,019), test (4,094), problem (3,892), condition (3,479), general (3,452), thanks (2,870), bladder (2,611), attention (2,518), carried (2,382), bowel (2,348), quality (1,520), professionalism (1,396), period (1,336), myeloma (1,306), removal (1,298), kidney (1,258), successful (854), endoscopy (846)

In addition to using statistical measures, a further step the researchers implemented was to remove keywords that occurred less than 50 times per million words (PMW) in both corpora. This step helped filter out those keywords that denoted proper nouns and sex-specific types of cancer, as well as the treatments associated with these. It should also be noted that CQPweb counts punctuation marks as tokens (and thus as potential keywords), which is why a bracket was key for the male patients' comments.

The researchers then closely analysed the keywords in order to identify their main functions in the feedback and whether and how these might relate to the patients' sex identities. To do this, they used the concordance view to access the uses of each keyword within its wider textual contexts and usually accessed entire comments when interpreting the keywords' functions. For keywords that occurred more than 100 times, the researchers analysed 100 randomly sampled cases.

Analysing these keywords, the researchers were able to identify a series of differences in the language used by male and female patients. The keyness of the generic illness-referring nouns *condition* and *problem* in the male patients' comments indicated a pronounced focus in these texts on the particular health issues that caused male patients to have to visit a provider. By analysing these words within their contexts of use, the researchers found that the male patients used them to characterise their care in terms of processes, of which they, their bodies and their health problems were the objects. This also helped to account for the keywords *carried*, *blood*, *endoscopy*, *removal* and *test*. Here is an example:

> My **condition** was discussed after a series of **blood tests** for diabetes, prostate **problems** and erectile dysfunction.

---

[1] Note that these keywords ranked as the top 30 when ordered according to the log likelihood scores assigned to them. For statistical information about the keywords, see Baker and Brookes (2022: 18–19).

Medical staff were often presented as performing the procedures that the male patients underwent, and could be indexed through uses of the keywords *general*, *hospital*, and *NHS*, which constituted a kind of metonymic reference whereby the male patients presented the performance of a few individual staff members in terms of representing an entire hospital or even the health system as a whole.

> Very happy with all aspects of treatment I have received from the **NHS**. Very impressed.

Rhetorically, this kind of reference has the potential to present the patient's experiences as applying not just to them or the individual staff members who treated them, but to staff comprising an entire hospital, the wider healthcare system and potentially other patients.

The male patients' comments also exhibited a marked use of words quantifying time (e.g., *months*, *period*), which tended to be used to quantify the amounts of time that the male patients had to wait for (typically) diagnoses and appointments.

> The first thing to do on entering the department was always to look at the screen to whether there were any delays. These often changed mainly to extend the waiting **period** up to 1 hour.

This attention to detail also helps account for the male patients' marked use of brackets, which they use to specify details such as the type of cancer they received treatment for, the type of treatment or procedures they underwent, and the ward or unit they received treatment on.

> Too many hospitals were involved ([name of hospital and ward]) in my opinion this resulted in months of inactivity and delay.

A somewhat curious set of keywords, also reflective of style, are the words *no*, *thanks* and *yes*. Rather than reflecting how the male patients linguistically performed evaluation, these words arose as key because of the way these patients interacted with the feedback form. In particular, the male patients interacted almost dialogically with the voice of the feedback form, answering the prompt questions literally (*no*, *yes*) and performing the speech act of thanking service providers, who were assumed to be represented by the voice of the form.

> **Yes**. It was dealt with in a timely fashion and consideration was given by the consultant for the eventual cosmetic appearance of the site following removal of the lesion.

> Just **thanks** for keeping me alive!

To account for this trend, the researchers considered another factor: age. They looked at the frequencies of the keywords *no*, *thanks* and *yes* by male and female patients at different ages. They found that the use of these terms

6.2 Using Demographic Metadata

increased with age, and their qualitative analysis of these words by patients at different age groups confirmed that this more dialogic style and literal interpretation of the prompt questions framing the free text boxes was indeed a feature more typical of older patients, particularly those over the age of 65 (see Baker and Brookes, 2022: 24). It could be the case that younger patients were more accustomed to the (synthetic) personalisation of such public discourse, rather than regarding it as an attempt by the organisation to establish personal dialogue. Importantly, by looking at the wider set of demographic metadata available to them, the researchers also found that the male patients featured were, on average, older than the female patients represented in the corpus. For example, male patients aged 75–84 contributed 22.42 per cent of all the words in the male patients' comments overall (compared to just 8.06 per cent contributed by this age group in the female patients' comments), while male patients aged 85+ contributed 3.9 per cent of all the words in the male patients' comments (compared to 1.45 per cent contributed by this age group in the female patients' comments). Thus, the researchers concluded that the keyness of these items was a product of the socio-demographic make-up of the corpus, with the sample of male patients represented within it being older, on average, than the sample of female patients.

Keywords for the female patients' comments were then obtained by comparing these against the male patients' comments. The resulting keywords, which are shown in the following list, were obtained in the same way as the male patients' keywords seen earlier.[2]

I (302,785), had (73,119), me (63,423), they (39,214), when (31,967), you (31,028), n't (29,681), so (28,576), chemotherapy (24,365), did (21,234), nurse (20,478), caring (18,756), feel (16,105), felt (13,101), radiotherapy (12,972), unit (11,739), kind (11,074), she (10,403), wait (10,315), everyone (9,969), oncologist (7,901), wonderful (7,106), her (6,637), amazing (6,436), chemo (6,056), supportive (4,998), busy (4,188), husband (3,164), lovely (2,961), lump (2,183)

While the male patients' comments focused characteristically on procedural and transactional aspects of service, the female patients tended to discursively situate themselves within their comments (as reflected, e.g., in the keywords *I* and *me*). This more personalised focus also gave rise to a discussion of the emotional impacts that the female patients' experiences had on them (as indicated in uses of the keywords *felt* and *feel*). Other keywords in the female patients' comments provide further evidence for this focus on interpersonal aspects of care, as staff members are evaluated using keywords such as *kind*, *lovely*, *supportive*, and *caring*.

---

[2] For statistical information about the keywords, see Baker and Brookes (2022: 18–19).

92   6 Language Use and Identity

The pronounced focus on interpersonal skills in the female patients' comments also gave rise to a stronger focus on individuals (*she, oncologist, her, nurse*), including the roles and experiences of relatives (*husband*), and units and smaller teams of staff (*they, unit*). Meanwhile, the keywords *chemotherapy, radiotherapy* and *chemo*, while referring ostensibly to types of treatment, were also used to refer to teams of staff (including metonymically through references to specific wards).

> The nurses in the **chemo** ward were absolutely fantastic at [name] Unit.

Therefore, while the male patients tended to present their evaluations as relevant to entire hospitals and the wider healthcare system, the female patients tended to focus on individuals or, at the most, small teams.

The keyword *everyone* was found to be frequently used in reference to other patients who attend a particular provider. The researchers interpreted this as a rhetorical strategy whereby the female patients rendered their experiences as more generalisable. A similar strategy these patients used to this end was to use the general *you*.

> **Everyone** is looked after in the same wonderful way.

> All staff in the cancer care unit are friendly, caring and helpful. They all welcome **you** and take care of **you** as if **you** are a part of the family.

Like the male patients, the female patients also focused on the theme of waits, as indicated in the keyword *wait*. However, the female patients were found to describe and evaluate waits in less-precise terms than the male patients (specifying the duration of their waits in just 15 per cent of cases). This was why the words *months* and *period* were key for the male patients' comments compared to the female patients', even if both groups focussed on waits in their feedback.

> Sometimes I have a long **wait** on surgery day but I don't think this can be helped.

In summary, by using socio-demographic metadata to annotate their corpus, then, Baker and Brookes (2022) were able to use the keywords technique to compare comments from the male and female patients represented in their data. This comparison revealed some differences in terms of the thematic content of the comments and what male and female patients focussed on or foregrounded within their feedback, finding, for example, that where male patients focussed on transactional aspects of care (e.g., operations), female patients tended to focus more on the people involved in their care, as well as the interpersonal relationships they established with staff. Moreover, analysis of the keywords also indicated how even shared areas of focus (e.g., waits) could be described and evaluated using characteristically different types of language, which involved providing differing levels of detail around those waits. Baker and

Brookes's (2022) study also demonstrated the value in having a wider set of demographic metadata tags to draw on for the purposes of interpreting patterns. In particular, they observed how male patients tended to engage in a more dialogic way with the feedback form than female patients did, and that this resulted in a markedly frequent use of words such as 'yes', 'no', and 'thanks', which functioned to answer the rhetorical prompt questions that framed the free text boxes. By drawing on metadata relating to patient age, the authors were able to conclude that this was likely to be an age effect, with older patients exhibiting this dialogic style more than younger ones. Thus, the authors argued that the (on average) older sample of male patients represented in their corpus was likely to be the reason for this difference. Without this wider demographic metadata, the authors might have concluded that this pattern was related to sex identity, rather than being down to a (likely) intersection of sex and age.

6.3 Using Mentions of Identity in the Data

The availability of reliable demographic metadata can, as the previously provided case study demonstrates, prove useful for organising corpus data for the purposes of studying identity. However, such metadata is not always available to us as analysts, particularly when we are studying language produced in anonymised contexts, such as many forms of online communication and social media. In such cases, if we are interested in studying the relationship between language use and identity, we must find another way of 'identifying the identities' of the language users represented in our data. One way we can do this is by using the language in the data itself, and looking for cases where language users openly disclose the particular aspects of their identity that we are interested in studying. Baker and co-authors (2019) employed this same approach. This study, which was a predecessor to that described in the previous section, involved a comprehensive analysis of the language of online patient feedback about a wide range of areas of healthcare provision in England (i.e., not just cancer services, as was the focus of Baker and Brookes's (2022) study). Their analysis was based on 228,113 online patient comments (28,971,412 words), posted to the NHS Choices website between 2013 and 2015.

6.3.1 Identifying Mentions of Sex Identity in a Corpus

As in the later study by Baker and Brookes (2022), Baker and co-authors (2019) undertook analyses that were designed to answer a series of questions that were put to them by their stakeholder partners in the NHS (see Chapter 2). As in the other study, here the stakeholder partners were also interested in learning about how patients' identities, including their sex identities, might influence the kind of feedback they gave and the language they used for their feedback. However, unlike in the other study, the set of patients' comments available to Baker and co-authors (2019) did not contain demographic metadata, since the online form through which patients posted their comments did not provide the facility through which such information could be provided. As such, to analyse the influence of patients' sex on the comments, Baker and co-authors (2019) searched for instances where patients mentioned their sex identity. In this way, they explored how sex identity categories 'cropped up', were 'oriented to' or otherwise 'noticed' by patients in their comments. This approach was broadly inspired by the approaches to 'membership categories' (Sacks, 1995) and 'person reference forms' (Schegloff, 1996) in conversation analysis, and offered the practical advantage of allowing the analysts to study how issues such as patients' sex identity figure in the comments, despite the absence of demographic metadata.

To find instances in which patients mentioned their sex identity, the analysts searched the corpus of comments for stretches of text in which either of the words *be*, *is*, *are*, *was* or *were* was followed by *man* or *woman* within the next five words (see also Chapter 2). This search yielded 518 cases for *man* and 332 for *woman*. Not all results actually involved cases where patients identified their own sex identity, as sometimes they could refer to that of another person (e.g., 'My GP is a good man'). Once such cases were removed, the analysts then took 200 cases (at random) for male self-identifiers and another 200 cases for female self-identifiers.

6.3.2 *Analysis of Language and Sex Identity Based on the Mention of Identity*

Baker and co-authors (2019) carried out various kinds of analyses on the resulting four hundred comments, including generating sets of keywords by comparing the comments from the male self-identifiers against the female ones, and vice versa. Tables 6.3 and 6.4 show, respectively, the keywords for the male and female patients' comments when these are compared against each other. Note that rather than take the top keywords from each list, by using relatively small samples of comments for this portion of their analysis, Baker and co-authors (2019) were able analyse all keywords produced through these comparisons (they considered all keywords that occurred at least 10 times and received a log likelihood score of at least 15.13, $p < 0.0001$.).

Keywords for male patients' comments compared to female patients' comments, ranked by frequency (in brackets)

the (1,688), of (543), have (484), this (343), you (262), been (189), appointment (157), practice (133), years (104), always (79), good (70), dentist (61), old (60), year (58), male (57), NHS (57), times (50), problem (48), given (47), many (45), helpful (43), minutes (34), condition (33), advice (29), men (28), poor (25), working (25), dental (25), wife (23), difficult (22), three (22), number

6.3 Using Mentions of Identity in the Data

(20), seems (18), surgeries (16), results (16), write (15), consultation (15), referral (15), non (13), following (13), bipolar (13), allowed (12), money (12), visits (12), recent (11), pains (11), five (10), doubt (10), surely (10)

Keywords for female patients' comments compared to male patients' comments, ranked by frequency (in brackets)

i (1,994), and (1,379), was (734), my (697), me (478), they (461), on (288), am (249), woman (153), after (139), hospital (110), said (89), never (83), did (75), life (63), ward (58), female (53), experience (53), first (53), didn't (50), her (45), baby (43), room (40), came (40), husband (39), lady (31), birth (31), pregnant (31), couldn't (30), women (29), around (29), lovely (29), wonderful (26), pregnancy (25), midwife (24), labour (21), grateful (20), midwives (18), amazing (17), impressed (17), nice (17), breast (15), crying (14), elderly (14), antibiotics (14), notes (13), booked (13), broken (11), drs (10), appt (10)

Unsurprisingly, the keywords show that female patients are more likely to use female-marked terms (usually when talking about themselves) and pregnancy, while male patients are more likely to use male-marked terms. Perhaps more interestingly, Baker and co-authors (2019) point out the differences in pronoun use. Female patients have a wider range of personal pronoun keywords and are more likely to use first-person forms (e.g., *me, my, I*). These tended to be used to describe personal experiences, often within narratives.

> Since there was no available appointments for **me**, **I** had to take a phone call consultation which **I** didn't mind. **They** told **me** to bring in a urine sample and **they** would leave the antibiotics with the receptionist.

The only pronoun keyword for the male patients was *you*. This tended to be used by the male patients to present their own experiences, but in a more impersonal way. This keyword was used regularly with the conditional *if* as a way of both addressing the presumed reader of the comment and making the attested experience appear more generalisable.

> If **you** call when the switchboard opens more often than not the line is engaged.

This use of the generalisable *you* by the male patients supports Charteris-Black and Seale's (2010: 64–5) observation that male patients tend to use more second-person pronouns than female patients, which they hypothesise is intended to 'make their accounts seem less personal and more objective and generalizable'. The patterns in personal pronoun usage suggested by the keywords listed indeed suggest different stereotypical strategies in terms of the ways that male and female patients compose their feedback, with some female patients being more likely to describe their experience in personal terms and some male patients attempting instead to impersonalise and accordingly generalise their narratives.

Another key difference identified by Baker and co-authors (2019) concerned the use of adjectives, especially those used in the explicitly evaluative aspects of feedback. Female patients' key evaluative adjectives included *lovely*, *nice*, *wonderful*, and *amazing*. Adjectives such as *lovely* and *nice* were argued to give a general impression of positive evaluation, but the authors also point out that they can be used in so many contexts that they eventually lose their meaning (becoming semantically 'empty'), especially if they are used frequently.

> I love this practice and can't sing its praises enough, the doctors, nurses and reception staff are all **nice** the practice management are **lovely** and always speaks or acknowledges.

An interesting keyword for the male patients is *pains*. Baker and co-authors (2019) point out that the word 'pain' can either be a count or a non-count noun, where saying we 'feel pain' is a non-count use but saying we 'feel a pain' is a count use, as it makes the pain a countable entity. The authors argue that when male patients discuss pain they are perhaps more likely to use the count, plural form as a way of emphasising the severity of their pain in order to legitimise their complaint without violating the gendered assumption that men should not feel pain, or at least the expectation that they should not usually complain about it (see also Jaworska and Ryan, 2018).

> I recently have called many times to make an appointment about my arm **pains**

Another notable difference indicated in the keywords is that the male patients are more likely to use words denoting time and quantification (i.e., *times*, *always*, *years*, *year*, *minutes*, *recent*, *many*, *three*, *five*, *number*). In some cases, a single comment could involve a rather intense use of such quantification, as in the following example:

> They **always** take between 20 to 40 **minutes** to speak with someone. Compare [Anonymised] to my previous surgeries this is at least 5 times faster. You should **always** remember a surgery has thousands of people registered and only a couple of administrators looking after it. If 10 people call at the same time you will have to wait for the 2 people working to get through them, which will take about 5 **minutes** a call, so 25 **minutes** if you were number 10!

Baker and co-authors (2019) interpret comments like this as representing a pronounced use of quantification rhetoric (see also Potter et al., 1991). They suggest that it constitutes another strategy and seems to represent yet another way in which some male patients sought to lend legitimacy and credibility to their complaints, while at the same time strengthening the impact of their feedback. For instance, in this example, the use of quantification rhetoric renders the feedback more specific and accurate (and thus more compelling) and helps emphasise the amount of inconvenience this patient experienced. Charteris-Black and Seale (2010) similarly observed that men tend to quantify and use numbers more often than female patients when talking about health and illness, a feature which they trace to the adoption of a traditionally masculine discourse style, arguing that 'men following traditional masculine styles have a discursive orientation to measuring and counting entities and processes rather than talking directly about what is happening to their own bodies' (2010: 71).

6.4 Conclusion

In this chapter we have considered two broad approaches to studying identity in a corpus of health communication data: one in which we can rely on demographic metadata tags and another in which we instead rely on cases where language users mention aspects of their identities in the language they produce. We focussed on two case studies which compared the language used by male and female patients in feedback given on healthcare services, with each study representing each of these approaches. Both approaches were helpful, in the sense that they allowed the analysts to organise and subsequently analyse their data in a manner that revealed interesting differences which the authors linked to differences in the performance of gender identities at the discursive level.

Patients' identities and the ways they construct these in their comments were found to have ramifications for how they evaluated healthcare services, including the types of linguistic strategies they used to frame this evaluation, contextualise their perspectives and legitimise their arguments. Interestingly, although both studies used quite different approaches, we can nevertheless observe some similarities in their findings. For example, among other things, both studies found that female patients tended to employ a more personalised style of feedback, while male patients tended to draw more on numbers and quantification. This suggests that some of the patterns reported across both studies are likely to be features of feedback in general, while also reflecting broader distinctions in the discourses associated with performances of particular gender identities. At the same time, the similarities in findings could be viewed as a kind of methodological triangulation; since these findings, which could apply to patient feedback as a genre in general, were arrived at through separate methodological routes, we can perhaps be more confident about their validity.

This point notwithstanding, either approach was also found to present certain advantages but also disadvantages, relative to the other. The annotation-based approach, although resource-intensive due to the need to annotate a large corpus with socio-demographic metadata, offers clear advantages in providing comprehensive insights into the socio-demographic balance of the corpus. Moreover, annotating a corpus with reliable demographic metadata permits the subsequent analysis of differences (and similarities) in language use among people from different identity-based backgrounds, at scale. An obvious advantage of this is that findings can be supported with statistical evidence, thus rendering them more robust and potentially more generalisable to the populations or healthcare contexts under study. However, a challenge of the approach is that it can create the trap of oversimplifying identity by relying on broad socio-demographic categories, potentially leading to us overlooking nuanced types of identity relations. Another notable limitation is the potential misinterpretation of statistically significant correlations as *causal* relationships, which might lead to us obscuring from our analytical gaze the possible influence of other aspects of language users' identity, in favour of focusing only on statistically significant trends.

The alternative approach, which involves relying on mentions of identity by language users in the language they produce, brings the advantage that we, as analysts, can perhaps be more confident that the aspects of identity we are focusing on to explain a linguistic pattern are indeed relevant to that pattern (since the language users invoke this themselves in their discourse). In other words, we can be more confident that an aspect of identity is relevant, as the language user has made it relevant by invoking it in their discourse. However, this approach also has several limitations, perhaps foremost being the relatively small amounts of data it is likely to give us (indeed, Baker et al. (2019) were only able to compare 200 texts each for male and female patients, from a corpus of more than 228,000 texts). The likely small sizes of samples obtained this way can restrict our analytical optionality (e.g., in terms of statistical measures available to us). Moreover, it can pose issues regarding data representativeness, both in terms of how far we can generalise on the basis of such small datasets, as well as what texts sampled in this way actually represent. In other words, we should ask: do texts in which people mention their identity represent a particular sort of language use, and can this be generalised to the wider population under study? The answer to this question will likely depend on the kind of language use being studied but should be considered critically if we are to take this kind of approach to sampling texts.

In view of the kinds of issues discussed previously, Baker and Brookes (2022) suggest that the most robust approach to studying identity in a corpus might be a mixed one which involves combining both of the approaches explored in this chapter. They suggest that this could involve assembling a large, demographically annotated corpus (where possible), but using the kind of approach based on cases where patients mention their identity (utilised by Baker et al. (2019)) to identify aspects of identity that are relevant to the kind of discourse and context under study, which can then be subjected to larger scale, quantitative analysis. Importantly, they stress that such an approach could help not only in identifying which aspects of identity are deemed relevant to the language users themselves but also support the interpretation of observed patterns and help account for the role of intersectional aspects of identity in a more data-driven way (i.e., by looking at the interaction of different aspects of identity because language users have evoked these themselves, rather than merely creating intersectional categories just because we have the demographic metadata available to us to do so).

References

Baker, P. (2010). *Sociolinguistics and Corpus Linguistics*. Edinburgh University Press.
　(2014). *Using Corpora to Analyze Gender*. Bloomsbury.
Baker, P. and Brookes, G. (2021). Lovely Nurses, Rude Receptionists, and Patronising Doctors: Determining the Impact of Gender Stereotyping on Patient Feedback. In J. Angouri and J. Baxter (eds.), *The Routledge Handbook of Language, Gender, and Sexuality* (pp. 559–71). Routledge.
　(2022). *Analysing Language, Sex and Age in a Corpus of Patient Feedback: A Comparison of Approaches*. Cambridge University Press.
Baker, P., Brookes, G. and Evans, C. (2019). *The Language of Patient Feedback: A Corpus Linguistic Study of Online Health Communication*. Routledge.
Benwell, B. and Stokoe, E. (2006). *Discourse and Identity*. Edinburgh University Press.
Burr, V. (2004). *Social Constructionism*, 2nd ed. Routledge.
Charteris-Black, J. and Seale, C. (2010). *Gender and the Language of Illness*. Palgrave Macmillan.
Coulter, A. (2006). Can Patients Assess the Quality of Health Care? *British Medical Journal*, *333*, 1–2. https://doi.org/10.1136/bmj.333.7557.1.
　(2013). Understanding the Experience of Illness and Treatment. In S. Ziebland, A. Coulter, J. D. Calabrese and L. Locock (eds.), *Understanding and Using Health Experiences: Improving Patient Care* (pp. 6–15). Oxford University Press.
Dunning, T. (1993). Accurate Methods for the Statistics of Surprise and Coincidence. *Computational Linguistics*, *19*(1), 61–74. Available at https://aclanthology.org/J93-1003.
Gleason, P. (1983). Identifying Identity: A Semantic History. *Journal of American History*, *69*(4), 910–31. https://doi.org/10.2307/1901196.
Graham, C. and Woods, P. (2013). Patient Experience Surveys. In S. Ziebland, A. Coulter, J. D. Calabrese and L. Locock (eds.), *Understanding and Using Health Experiences: Improving Patient Care* (pp. 81–93). Oxford University Press.
Habermas, J. (1975). Moral Development and Ego Identity. *Telos, 1975*(24), 41–55. https://doi.org/10.3817/0675024041.
Hardie, A. (2012). CQPweb: Combining Power, Flexibility and Usability in a Corpus Analysis Tool. *International Journal of Corpus Linguistics*, *17*(3), 380–409. https://doi.org/10.1075/ijcl.17.3.04har.
　(2014). *Log Ratio: An Informal Introduction*. Online. http://cass.lancs.ac.uk/log-ratio-an-informal-introduction/. Accessed 16 May 2023.

Jaworska, S. and Ryan, K. (2018). Gender and the Language of Pain in Chronic and Terminal Illness: A Corpus-Based Discourse Analysis of Patients' Narratives. *Social Science & Medicine*, *215*, 107–14. https://doi.org/10.1016/j.socscimed.2018.09.002.

Leech, G. (1997). Introducing Corpus Annotation. In R. Garside, G. Leech and T. McEnery (eds.), *Corpus Annotation: Linguistic Information from Computer Text Corpora* (pp. 1–18). Routledge.

Potter, J., Wetherell, M. and Chitty, A. (1991). Quantification Rhetoric – Cancer on Television. *Discourse and Society*, *2*(3), 333–65. https://doi.org/10.1177/0957926591002003005.

Preece, S. (2016). Introduction: Language and Identity in Applied Linguistics. In S. Preece (ed.), *The Routledge Handbook of Language and Identity* (pp. 1–16). Routledge.

Sacks, H. (1995). *Lectures on Conversation: Volumes 1 and 2*. Blackwell.

Schegloff, E. A. (1996). Some Practices for Referring to Persons in Talk-in-Interaction: A Partial Sketch of a Systematics. In A. Fox (ed.), *Studies in Anaphora* (pp. 437–85). John Benjamins.

Sinclair, J. M. (1992). The Automatic Analysis of Corpora. In J. Svartvik (ed.), *Directions in Corpus Linguistics: Proceedings of the Nobel Symposium 82* (pp. 379–97). Mouton De Gruyter.

Vingerhoets, E., Wensing, M. and Grol R. (2001). Feedback of Patients' Evaluations of General Practice Care: A Randomised Trial. *BMJ Quality & Safety*, *10*, 224–8. https://doi.org/10.1136/qhc.0100224.

7 Change over Time

7.1 Introduction

Language is not static, and one of the benefits of corpus linguistics has been to identify changes in language use over time. For example, Leech and colleagues (2009) and Baker (2017) have compared matched sets of written corpora which point to a set of major changes in English that could be characterised as densification (fitting increased information into less space), democratisation (avoidance of signalling hierarchies or prejudiced references to others), and informalisation (language which replicates features of informal face-to-face communication).

It can be useful to consider change over time within corpora relating to health as a way of revealing emerging linguistic patterns that can indicate new ways of conceptualising health conditions. A time-based analysis may also be able to show the impact on language of a key event such as the passage of a piece of health legislation or the availability of a new form of medication or therapy. In this chapter we will focus on three case studies of corpora relating to change over time – changing representations of obesity in newspapers, changes in patient feedback over time, and changes in language use about anxiety on an online forum.

Corpus approaches are well-suited for identifying a range of aspects of language change, as a wide number of features can be taken into account at once, and statistical tests will identify those which show the most impressive changes. Such approaches require the collection of texts from multiple points in time. Most corpus tools enable two corpora to be compared together easily, via the keywords technique, and if such texts are from different time periods and constitute matched sources, it would be possible to make claims about increases or decreases of a particular feature, although it should be borne in mind that a comparison of a small number of sampling points (e.g., two or three) does not allow us to express confidence that we are seeing a trend. In particular, if the sampling points are not from adjacent time periods (e.g., texts from only the years 1980 and 2000), we are essentially looking at 'snapshots' in time, and any observed increases or decreases may obscure a more complex picture if data had been collected from, say, 1985, 1990, and 1995.

An important question to consider when carrying out a corpus analysis of change over time is how to divide the corpora into time periods. There are a number of criteria to bear in mind. First, are there any significant events which would suggest that the corpus could be segmented into meaningful sections? Second, how many sections should be compared? Depending on the amount of text available, splitting data into numerous sections is likely to result in lower frequencies of many linguistic phenomena, meaning that it can be difficult to have confidence about whether differences in frequency are actually meaningful or due to chance. Third, how long should each time period cover? Studies could compare centuries, decades, years, months, weeks, or even days. However, there needs to be a reasonably clear justification for the length of time that is used to delineate the sub-corpus segments. This decision should be related to the data under consideration. In some contexts, language use around a health-related topic might develop very quickly, whereas in others, the pace may be very slow. For many health-related news topics, taking a corpus consisting of a year's worth of articles and then comparing each month may not reveal much, unless there was a highly significant event relating to the topic during that year. Having segments that are too broad may make important aspects of change difficult to identify. For example, comparing corpora of nineteenth- and twentieth-century texts about mental illness against one another might risk obscuring the broad changes in perceptions of mental health that have occurred, especially in the twentieth century.

7.2 Patient Feedback: Identifying Increasing and Decreasing Lexical Items over Time

The first case study discussed in this chapter involves patient feedback. The NHS sends an annual survey to all patients who had received treatment relating to a diagnosis of some form of cancer. These surveys contain questions with sets of predetermined answers which patients can respond to by ticking a box, as well as three questions which allow patients to write their own answers as text. Thus, patients were asked 'Was there anything good about your NHS cancer care?', 'Was there anything that could be improved?', and 'Any other comments?'. The answers to these three questions comprised our corpus. As the researchers had been given the answers to surveys sent out in 2015–18, there were four years of language data to compare.

Corpus tools are somewhat less developed for comparisons of multiple corpora, although it is possible to carry out workarounds using the keywords method (see Section 7.3) or to use a measure called the coefficient of variation, or CV (Figure 7.1; Baker, 2017: 61–2), which essentially takes the mean of the

7.2 Patient Feedback

$$Cv = \left(\frac{\sigma}{\mu}\right) 100$$

Figure 7.1 The coefficient of variation.

relative frequencies of a linguistic item across three or more time-linked corpora (σ), divides it by the standard deviation of the item (μ), and multiples by 100. A high CV (close to 100) indicates an item which shows a great deal of variation across the corpora, whereas a low CV (close to 0) indicates items that have remained fairly stable in frequency over time.

The CV was used to compare lexical change over time across the 4 years of patient feedback. To identify the most important trends the researchers focussed on a set of high frequency words, stipulating that a word must occur at least 500 times in one of the time periods under examination in order to be considered for analysis. This resulted in a set of 721 lexical items. In order to identify candidate words, their total frequencies, and their individual frequencies across each of the 4 years, WordSmith Tools (Scott, 2016) was used, being one of the most efficient corpus analysis tools for creating tables of multiple wordlists. First, individual wordlists for each (sub-)corpus were created. Then the option 'Detailed Consistency' was selected from the 'Getting Started' menu within the 'WordList' tool, and the four wordlists were chosen in order to obtain word frequencies for each corpus. This data was then exported into Microsoft Excel. In Excel, researchers first needed to calculate the relative frequencies of each word (for this study, occurrences per million words was used). Then the CVs for each word were calculated. This involved calculating the standard deviation for the standardised frequency of each word (the STDEV function in Excel), dividing this by the average of each word (AVERAGE function), and then multiplying by 100. If the frequencies of the four wordlists were given in columns B, C, D, and E in an Excel spreadsheet, then the formula to calculate the CV would be as follows:

=STDEV(B2:E2)/AVERAGE(B2:E2)*100

The words were then ordered according to their CV score and the words with the highest CVs which also showed a *constant* increase or decrease over time were identified. For example, *ongoing* has a frequency profile of 101.5, 102.2, 180.9, and 185.8 occurrences per million words over the 4 years – with each relative frequency being higher than the one before it – whereas *food* shows a constantly decreasing profile (554.5, 470.7, 453.5, and 405.0). These words, along with their relative frequencies and CVs, are shown in Table 7.1.

Table 7.1 *Constantly increasing and decreasing high-frequency words over time in patient feedback*

	2015	2016	2017	2018	CV
Constantly increasing over time					
ongoing	101.5	102.2	180.9	185.8	32.90
follow-up	108.9	116.1	127.8	193.1	28.23
amazing	397.0	502.2	616.2	709.6	24.22
administration	174.1	220.6	248.6	282.3	19.77
NHS	1,523.4	1,738.7	1,835.0	2,054.5	12.09
process	232.2	252.5	285.1	304.8	12.00
journey	117.9	132.2	145.2	156.3	11.71
outstanding	287.0	320.5	351.3	377.6	11.19
none	294.0	277.4	333.9	354.0	10.92
cancelled	139.6	159.7	145.8	178.0	10.92
knowledgeable	120.2	114.7	123.8	144.7	10.43
grateful	497.8	550.5	609.3	628.2	10.36
compassionate	118.5	121.0	140.4	144.7	10.16
plan	147.6	161.1	167.2	188.0	10.13
issues	147.0	153.9	163.8	164.7	10.12
stage	227.4	216.5	244.3	269.6	9.57
Constantly decreasing over time					
food	554.5	470.7	453.5	405.0	13.22
wards	317.7	280.2	269.1	239.3	11.72
night	451.2	438.0	377.3	370.4	10.09
visits	249.7	235.7	227.4	197.1	9.77
drugs	263.0	236.8	222.0	211.1	9.63
attitude	227.1	219.3	204.9	185.0	8.84
ward	2,037.6	1,932.8	1,761.1	1,676.8	8.81

The words in Table 7.1 were then subjected to a more detailed qualitative analysis, via samples of concordance lines (random samples of 100 lines for each word for each year were analysed), to try to identify their most typical uses and whether their uses had changed over time. A few illustrative findings from the analysis are given as follows.

Some of the increasing words indicate specific ways of making positive evaluations of staff that patients encountered (*amazing, outstanding, knowledgeable, compassionate*) and giving thanks (*grateful*). Additionally, the word *none* tended to be used in two ways, both of which were linked to positive evaluations. It often occurred in the phrase *second to none*, which was used in praise-giving. For example,

The care and treatment was **second to none**.

7.2 Patient Feedback

However, *none* also tended to occur on its own, and in more than 90 per cent of cases it was given as a short, explicit answer to the question 'Was there anything that could be improved?'

NHS also tended to occur in positive feedback, often to indicate support for the NHS as an institution, sometimes in comments that acknowledge or allude to threats around it or funding issues.

> Long live the **NHS**
>
> I get very annoyed when I hear or read about people 'bashing' the **NHS**
>
> With all the **NHS** cutbacks we hear about in the media I feel I was treated well and quickly

Some increasing words were used in mixed ways. For example, *journey* is another word which has increased over time. This word can refer to literal journeys (e.g., the journey from home to hospital and back again) or refer to the patient's experience with cancer as a metaphorical journey. When *journey* was used in negative feedback, it usually involved complaints about literal journeys.

> On follow up appointment there was no results given as they were inconclusive, it was a waste of 4 hour **journey**.

On the other hand, when *journey* was used in positive feedback, it tended to be metaphorical.

> I was given booklets and leaflets to help me through this very difficult **journey**

An increasing word that was used in more negative contexts was *cancelled*, which usually occurred in complaints about appointments or operations being cancelled.

> Operation **cancelled** once at end of one day waiting
>
> Called to appointment where appointment **cancelled** without notification

In terms of words that decreased over time, many of these tended to occur in the context of patients writing about overnight stays: *wards, ward, food, bed, night*. These words are all more likely to occur in negative as opposed to positive feedback, particularly *bed*. Complaints about beds include lack of a bed for patients, not being able to adjust beds, disturbances from patients in other beds, or being too cold in bed. Complaints relating to the word *night* involve lack of night staff or problems with night staff, patients having a poor night's sleep due to noise, or not getting home from appointments until late at night. The fact that such words have decreased over time would suggest that issues about overnight stays appear to have gradually improved between 2015 and 2018.

This study focussed on change in terms of words or lexical frequencies. However, it is possible to examine change in terms of other kinds of phenomena, such as fixed sequences of words (sometimes called lexical bundles or clusters) or part-of-speech categories. Tools like CLAWS7 (Constituent Likelihood Automatic Word-tagging System), which can be accessed through the online corpus analysis tool Wmatrix (Rayson, 2008), automatically classify the words in a corpus according to their part-of-speech, usually with accuracy rates of around 95–8 per cent. The system assigns a part-of-speech tag to each word from a predefined set of 137 tags (e.g., NN1 refers to a singular common noun while NN2 is a plural common noun). Considering changes over time in relation to frequencies of part-of-speech tags might enable researchers to identify patterns of language at the grammatical level as opposed to the lexical level.

In addition, Wmatrix assigns tags to words based on a set of semantic categories (using a second tagset called USAS), consisting of 21 higher-order tags which are subdivided into around 600 more fine-grained categories based on thesaurus definitions. For example, category G is 'Government and Public', while G2.1 is 'Law and Order' (consisting of words like *court*, *rules*, and *legal*) and G2.1 is 'Crime' (consisting of words like *evil*, *corruption*, and *guilt*). The system can be used to identify changing themes or topics across time-linked corpora, although care should be taken to ensure that words have been accurately assigned to categories, and in some cases, a more productive analysis might be one where the analyst has created their own categories and assigned relevant words to them. This would be useful in cases where the corpus contains lexis that the tagger does not recognise or assigns to inappropriate categories. Additionally, the categories in USAS may not fully capture the most meaningful semantic distinctions that the analyst wants to consider. USAS is able to recognise names of people but does not categorise them according to whether they are a politician, a sportsperson, or a news broadcaster, for example.

The CV approach to change over time tends to be more effective when there are three to five time periods to compare, and as noted earlier, it tends to work better when dealing with medium- to high-frequency phenomena (which is why comparing categories like grammatical tags can be productive). In the following section, we describe a different approach with more data collection points, where researchers created their own categorisation system (using a bottom-up approach), in order to examine changes in language over time relating to obesity.

7.3   Representations of Obesity: Identifying Changing Topics over Time and Considering the Annual News Cycle

In this section we discuss a project which involved examining representation around obesity in a 36-million-word corpus of British newspaper articles (see

7.3 Representations of Obesity

Chapters 2 and 3). The time span of this corpus was from 2008 to 2017, so the corpus contained a decade's worth of articles taken from 11 UK national newspapers. This data was initially analysed by splitting the corpus into 10 sub-corpora, each consisting of a year's worth of text. The analysis aimed to identify lexical items which had increased or decreased over time. In order to obtain a set of relevant terms, the whole corpus was compared against a reference corpus (in this case the 100-million-word British National Corpus), and a list of the top keywords was obtained. The relative frequencies of these keywords were then obtained for each of the 10 years of data, in order to identify words which had become more (or less) popular over time.

However, this resulted in a problem. The data across the 10 years of the newspaper corpus was not well-distributed. For example, in the year 2011, 2,564 articles were published, whereas 2016 had 6,734 articles. The vast majority of articles were published after 2013, meaning that when keywords were obtained from the whole corpus, the period from 2013 to 2017 greatly influenced the resulting list. The researchers wanted to take into account words that might have been keywords in the earlier part of the corpus, but many words did not appear as key because their frequencies were too low compared to the frequencies of words in the later time periods. To address this issue, it was decided to calculate keywords separately for each year of the corpus, by using a method called 'the remainder method'. This involves taking a year of data (e.g., 2008) and obtaining keywords from it, using the remainder of the corpus as the reference corpus (in this case the data from 2009 to 2017). This technique was then carried out for each year of the corpus separately, resulting in 10 keyword lists. The researchers then took the top-100 keywords from each list and merged them together. Some keywords appeared in multiple lists, so when these repetitions were removed, the list contained 745 distinct keywords.

At this point, the researchers carried out concordance analyses to group the keywords into meaningful categories. For example, one category created was called ILLNESS, and keywords like *cancer*, *diabetes*, and *inflammation* were placed in it. The keyword *heart* was also placed in this category. Even though it appears to refer to a body part, concordance analysis showed that it was almost always used to refer to heart attacks. Having identified 27 categories of words in this way, the collective relative frequencies of the words in the categories was calculated, for each of the 10 years of the corpus, and this was plotted as a chart.

Figure 7.2 shows the relative frequencies for the category FOOD, which consisted of keywords like *fruit*, *diet*, and *junk*. This can be created in Microsoft Word or Excel by entering the numbers into a chart. A trendline (shown as a dotted line) can also be automatically added, showing that in general the relative frequency of FOOD words has increased over time. The equation of the trendline is also shown in Figure 7.2. The higher the first number, the steeper

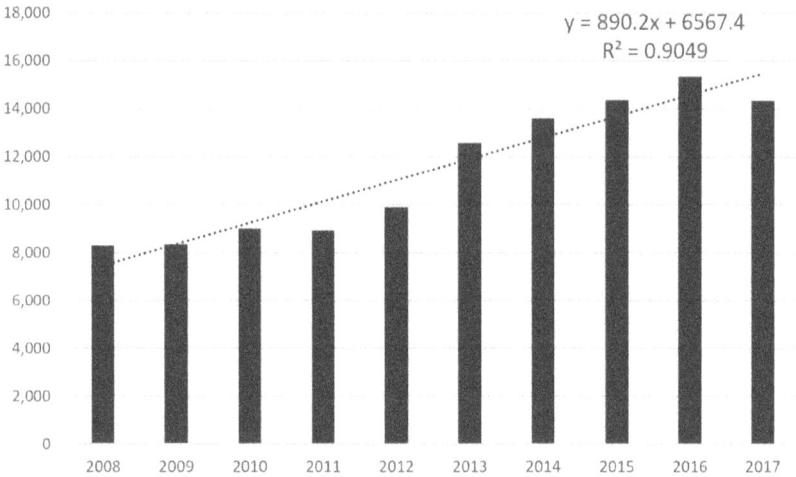

Figure 7.2 Relative frequencies of words categorised as FOOD over time in UK news articles about obesity.

the gradient and thus the more dramatic the change over time. The score of 890.2 was the steepest gradient of the 27 categories observed. The second number in the equation (6,567.4 in this case) indicates the 'intercept', the first point of the trendline on the graph (in this case for the year 2008). The R^2 value indicates how well the trendline fits the observed data, with a score of 1 being an exact fit. Here the R^2 is 0.9049, showing that the data is a very close fit to the trendline. Charts like this were created for all 27 categories.

Overall, the analysis found that two kinds of categories had increased over time. First, categories which framed obesity as due to personal responsibility had increased. This included FOOD, as we have seen, and another category called LIFESTYLE, which contained keywords like *sleep*, *tobacco*, and *gardening*. A second set of increasing categories referenced a biomedical explanatory model of obesity. This included the categories BIOLOGY (containing keywords like *genes*, *cells*, *testosterone*) and RESEARCH (*experts*, *findings*, *study*). Thus, excerpts like the following two tended to increase over time (and keywords are shown in bold typeface).

> The desire for **food** in obese people is associated with **brain** activity that 'rewards' their behaviour, in a similar manner to substance addicts, the research suggests. (*Mirror*, August 2015)

> Further **findings** showed participants who skipped breakfast were more likely to have an overall unhealthy **lifestyle**, including poor **diet**, frequent **alcohol** consumption and **smoking**. (*Express*, 2 October 2017)

7.3 Representations of Obesity

Categories which were decreasing over time included those labelled as SOCIAL (e.g., *inequality, unemployment, discrimination*), POLITICAL UK (e.g., *government, MPs, political*), BUSINESS (e.g., *market, profits, commercial*), and PLACES (NON-UK). The top category (having the lowest 'x' value) was PLACES UK (*Britain, London, UK*), often being used in contexts which compared statistics and policy around obesity in the UK with other countries, particularly involving news stories where the UK was described as not doing as well compared to other places. The following two excerpts show examples of keywords that were less likely to appear over time.

> A leaked draft revealed that the **government** had dropped a target to halve **childhood** obesity in ten years along with more stringent incentives to make the food **industry** act. (*Times*, 18 August 2017)

> Experts said many countries could learn from Scandanavian eating habits. Latest figures show obesity levels in **Denmark** are half those in **Britain**. In **Denmark**, 13.4 per cent of adults are obese, compared with 26.1 per cent in the **UK**. (*Telegraph*, 1 September 2014)

The analysis indicates that during the period under study, UK press framing of obesity tended to be increasingly placed at the level of the individual – either due to lifestyle choices or biological and genetic factors that impact on our likelihood of gaining weight. On the other hand, framing of obesity tended to move away from structural and social factors, relating to the roles of government or industry. Newspapers also focussed less on obesity policy in other countries, particularly when such policies appear to have resulted in a more successful outcome than in the UK.

In order to explain these findings, it is first worth considering that between 1993 and 2010, there was generally an increase in the percentage of people with obesity in the UK, but in the following decade, the proportion remained fairly stable (Baker, 2019: 4; Corrigan and Scarlett, 2020: 6; National Statistics, 2018: 2; Scottish Government, 2017: 4). Fifteen per cent of adults had obesity in 1993, whereas this figure was around 25 to 27 per cent between 2010 and 2016. So, in the UK, obesity was historically high but also fairly stable during the period under study. It is also worth making a connection between the government in power in the decade under examination. From 2008 to 2010, there was a Labour-run government. In 2010 this was replaced with a Conservative-led alliance with the Liberal Democrat Party, and in 2015 the Conservatives won an election outright and remained in power for the rest of the time period under study. Although the British press is independent, the majority of the newspapers in the corpus supported the Conservative government, which explains, to an extent, why articles around government policy towards obesity have tended to reduce over time, in favour of articles which focus on individual responsibility. This has the twin function of avoiding criticism of the government's role in failing to reduce high levels of obesity, while supporting the Conservative party's neo-liberal political goals that place more emphasis on the individual rather than social institutions to solve problems.

Both the patient feedback study (Section 7.2) and the press representation of obesity study (this section) considered change by comparing a set of sequential time periods (in this case each sub-corpus consisted of a single year of data). This method tends to be one of the most typical ways of looking at change over time, and depending on the time span that the data covers and the overall size of the corpus, we could make the sub-corpora represent smaller or larger periods of time accordingly. For example, if you have a corpus which covers 100 years of data, you might want to split the data into 10 decades or four periods of 25 years each. Another option would be to divide the data according to significant events. One way of dividing up the obesity news data, for example, could be into sections that denote the different governments mentioned previously.

However, there are other ways to consider change over time, and for the remainder of this chapter we will examine three other perspectives. First, remaining with the newspaper corpus on obesity, we could consider time in terms of the annual news cycle. If we consider a single year, there will be a series of events which can be predicted to an extent. For example, for the UK, there will be cooler temperatures in November through February while the period of June through August is likely to be warmer. Additionally, children are likely to be out of school around Christmas, Easter, and the month of August, meaning that many families will travel on holiday during those periods. There are also routines in terms of the political calendar – with the annual budget occurring in March while party conferences usually take place in the autumn season. To an extent, these kinds of events are fixed, occurring around the same time each year. As a result, we could think of change over time in relationship to annual cycles, and instead of comparing the different years in a corpus we could compare the different months against one another.

A keywords analysis, again using the remainder method, was thus carried out to derive 12 sets of keywords (1 for each month). The top-10 keywords for each month are shown in Table 7.2 (only 8 keywords were obtained for September). For a keyword to qualify as truly being associated with a particular month, it was stipulated that it needed to occur at least 100 times. All keywords which appeared at least half of the time in only a single year of the corpus were also removed. This was to avoid cases where a single news story dominated a particular point in time – such cases tended not to be true 'monthly' keywords, whereas the researchers wanted to focus on keywords which cropped up every year in the same month.

Concordance analyses of the keywords (shown in the following examples, in bold print) indicate how obesity tends to be framed differently throughout the year. For example, in January there is a focus on weight loss through dieting, along with losing weight as part of New Year's resolutions, whereas

7.3 Representations of Obesity

Table 7.2 *Monthly keywords for the 'Obesity in the News' corpus*

Month	Keywords
January	sugar, you, diet, resolutions, cubes, weight, eat, lose, food, calories
February	yoga, insomnia, sleep, asthma, profits, pollution, ambulance, alcohol, butter, welfare
March	sugar, chocolate, sleep, liver, announced, teaspoons, anorexia, sugary, price, gout
April	eggs, egg, dementia, underweight, gardening, BMI, teachers, teacher, chocolate, running
May	obesity, overweight, bacteria, gut, she, her, eating, vegan, study, salt
June	diabetes, babies, milk, corn, her, syrup, she, traffic, broccoli, girls
July	dementia, school, fertility, coconut, meals, pupils, sweeteners, pasta, society, park
August	sport, sports, sporting, antibiotics, I, cycling, brain, drugs, PE, swimming
September	school, your, uniform, pupils, risk, cook, link, diabetes, she, sleep
October	NHS, report, he, conference, health, patients, minister, care
November	walking, stress, funding, men, midwives, tax, birth, sleep, vitamin, soda
December	sales, mince, resolutions, turkey, pies, pudding, alcohol, discrimination, dementia, obese

in February and March, stories about lack of sleep being responsible for obesity tend to be more common.

> The **diet** has **you** eat foods that the medical literature suggests are good for the brain. (*Independent*, 6 January 2016)

> One in eight Brits **sleep** for less than six hours and **insomnia** has been linked to obesity, heart disease and cancer. (*The Sun*, 26 February 2013)

August has more stories relating to weight loss via participation in sports, perhaps as a result of good weather at this time of year.

> **Sports** like handball are fun, easy, cheap and social. If we can encourage children to do more **sport** at school, it will help them realise playing **sport** is fun, not boring. (*The Sun*, 7 August 2012)

October contains stories which relate obesity to government policy, as the news reports on speeches at party conferences.

> Tories blasted for railing against child obesity at party **conference** sponsored by a sugar firm. (*Mirror*, October 2017)

The analysis shows how different ways of framing obesity shift in and out of focus as a year progresses, with responsibility around obesity more likely to be placed at the personal level at certain times of year or linked to government policy at other points. The result is a somewhat inconsistent form of messaging, with suggestions around weight loss also fluctuating between different types or amounts of physical activity (sleeping in February, playing sports in August, walking in November) and/or dieting. It could be argued that an effective way of reducing obesity would be to follow a consistent routine, rather than putting one's metabolism and body under stress for short periods by engaging in periods of overeating followed by diets, or engaging in sporadic exercise routines which change across the year. One finding which emerged from this study is that the news cycle's imperative to continuously report new angles on a topic, coupled with seasonal trends, is perhaps likely to inadvertently hinder some people's efforts to lose weight.

Obviously, not every corpus study is going to reveal interesting differences as the result of annual cycles, and several years of corpus data would need to be available in order to gain a sense of the repetition of the cycle. We would encourage readers to think creatively when considering change over time, though, and in the final section of this chapter, we describe some other ways that change can be conceptualised.

7.4   Anxiety Forum: Age and Level of Experience as Types of Time

The third case study in this chapter involves two other ways of considering change over time, relating to a 21-million-word corpus of online forum posts about anxiety. These posts were made between 2012 and 2020, and one way which the researchers analysed change over time in the corpus was to consider how words and word categories increased or decreased from 1 year to the next, using techniques already described in the previous sections. However, they also considered change over time in two other ways. The first was to think about the age of the participants, while the second was to look at the length of time that a participant had been engaging with the forum. We will first consider the age of participants.

The vast majority of contributors to the forum only posted for a few months, so the age at the time they posted was fairly static. Therefore, the forum posts could be divided into different age groups and compared against one another. Here, change over time is conceived as being related to the age of each person who had contributed to the corpus (i.e., in the number of years).

When the researchers obtained the corpus data, it was accompanied by a substantial amount of metadata which had been derived from forum users' profile information, including sex, country of residence, ethnicity, and age. Not every person who created a profile provided information about all of these aspects, and for the category of age, only 56 per cent of forum users did so. Of those who did give their age, the majority were aged between 20 and 70. The researchers thus decided to reduce the corpus slightly, to consider posters between these two ages and then divide them into groups for comparison. Assigning people to age groups is an arbitrary practice, to an extent. This was done very simply, in terms of decades (e.g., 20s, 30s, 40s), in order to facilitate a manageable number of sub-corpora (six in total) for comparison. The

7.4 Anxiety Forum: Age and Level of Experience

remainder method, described earlier, was used to obtain keywords for each of these age groups. So, for the 20s age group, the posts of everyone aged 20–9 was compared against the posts made by everyone aged 30 and above, and this was done for each age group. Keywords were then examined through collocate and concordance analyses in order to group similar keywords into themes and to also gain a better impression regarding how each age group used the words under examination.

A potential issue with this approach related to prolific posters. A small number of posters tended to dominate the forum at different points in time, and their idiosyncratic uses of language resulted in large numbers of keywords appearing for each age group. While such keywords tell us something interesting about individual posters, it is not perhaps fair to say that they are *typical* of the language use of a particular time period or age group, so keywords that were used 50 per cent or more by a single poster were removed. Additionally, keywords that referred to people's usernames were removed. Many usernames had already been removed, through an automatic tool, prior to the researchers receiving the corpus, but some had escaped detection.

The analysis was carried out in Sketch Engine, and the 20 strongest keywords for each age group are shown in Table 7.3 (with the frequencies for that age group provided in brackets).

Table 7.3 *Top-20 keywords (and frequencies) for age-groups by decade in the 'Anxiety Forum' corpus*

Age	Keywords
20s	♥ (357), :((1,770), idk (639), yeah (1,187), wanna (584), boyfriend (591), scared (2,794), weird (1,423), gonna (902), guys (767), feels (2,098), die (1,192), thankyou (632), freaking (394), college (349), okay (1,219), haha (409), constantly (1,039), kinda (411), literally (627)
30s	:) (5,320), issue (959), allow (542), u (3,366), once (2,528), ur (752), headaches (1,022), ER (708), body (3,796), cycle (560), everyday (1,253), kids (911), dizzy (1,452), gotten (518), sensation (655), happen (1,911), medication (3,118), afraid (1,352), coming (1,507), while (2,573)
40s	oh (1,075), Sertraline (401), its (4,253), lol (1,422), etc (666), CBT (736), hi (5,365), Dr (702), kids (540), awful (788), dad (427), OK (1,610), yes (2,450), wow (313), mum (498), counselling (307), ive (812), u (1747), im (2,444), hugs (483)
50s	Mr (367), B12 (392), deficiency (227), xx (2,694), hey (441), menopause (163), wont (252), cant (629), thats (438), n (401), love (2,581), post (1,159), daughter (590), advise (270), anorexia (80), listen (524), welcome (586), members (190), apps (119), website (242)
60s	regards (311), wishes (394), site (749), xxxx (304), love (1,753), Venlafaxine (147), GP (1,002), evening (304), Klonopin (161), bless (328), pleased (178), husband (464), perhaps (252), counselling (261), posting (208), luck (871), lots (451), antidepressant (128), problems (826)

7 Change over Time

Subsequently, a more detailed concordance and collocates analysis of the keywords in Table 7.3 indicated that posters in their 20s tended to take on an advice-seeking role in the forum, and also tended to characterise their anxiety using much more extreme forms of language than older people.

> i just remember being in his car and it cold outside and just feeling like a little mouse in a trap. thats **literally** what i am, a little mouse and the world is the trap and i want out (20s)

> I **constantly** check my body in a mirror I have no clue how many times a day (20s)

> And the dreams make no sense at all or they're about what gives me anxiety then I'll wake up in the middle of the night **scared** and thinking I'm gonna **die**. (20s)

On the other hand, older posters tended to take on a more supportive, advice-giving role, although different forms of advice tended to be given, depending on the age of the poster: for example, those in their 30s were more likely to recommend different forms of medication, whereas those older than 40 tended to recommend counselling. There were differences in the ways that anxiety was conceived, with those in their 30s referring to *issues*, while people in their 60s talked about *problems*.

> Knowing your past focus on health **issues**, it sounds like an anxiety **issue**. (30s)

> Sounds like you've got **problems**? I hope you will be able to resolve them, but don't forget we are all here to help (60s)

This may appear like a 'cosmetic' difference, although it was found that across the whole corpus *issues* tended to collocate with words which had a discourse prosody for importance (*important, key, major, serious, critical*) and acknowledgement (*address, raise, discuss, facing*) rather than resolution, whereas *problems* tended to have a discourse prosody which suggested something had the capacity to be solved (*solve, solving, solved, solution, fix, address, resolve*). In order to further interpret and explain the findings, the full analysis (see Collins and Baker, 2023) went beyond the anxiety forum corpus to consider the ways that younger people use language more generally by consulting a spoken reference corpus, as well as taking into account recent societal developments such as the popularity of social media and various increasing pressures on young people.

Moving on to the final way that was considered, change over time related to the amount of time that a person has spent on the forum. In the anxiety forum, about a third of posters only made a single post, whereas almost 80 per cent made fewer than 10 posts and about 8 per cent made between 10 and 20 posts. About 12 per cent of posters made more than 20 posts.

It is interesting to consider how people's roles changed as they continued to interact with the forum, and how this might be reflected through their language use. Sub-corpora were therefore created of people's first, twentieth, fortieth,

7.4 Anxiety Forum: Age and Level of Experience

sixtieth, and final posts to the forum, and then keywords were derived and examined via concordance analyses. In order to identify changes in the 'journey' that people make as they interact with the forum, the sub-corpus containing the first posts that people made was compared against all of the other posts to derive keywords. This was also done for the 20th, 40th, 60th, and final posts that people made. (The keywords are shown in Table 7.4, with their frequencies in brackets.)

The qualitative analysis of keywords through concordancing found that posters initially sought advice and provided their personal histories.

> Does **anyone** know how I can get my life back? Be greatly **appreciated**. (1st post)

> hi everyone i am **new** here my **name** is x i am **male** from egypt 28 **years** and i think i have anxiety **since** i was 16. (1st post)

Table 7.4 *Keywords at various points in the forum posters' journey*

Post	Keywords
1st	recently (1,390), diagnosed (953), old (1,807), suffered (946), year (2,548), constantly (1,185), started (3,827), anyone (3,420), years (5,185), attacks (2,393), since (2,859), social (655), months (2,744), suffering (1,262), new (2,405), ago (2,760), severe (816), male (231), appreciated (339), almost (1,258), constant (845), can't (3,739), depression (2,067), sick (1,700), month (1,083), currently (566), past (1,576), female (222), joined (275), experiencing (640), school (823), extreme (360), similar (797), die (1,045), dying (766), extremely (475), attack (2,562), am (10,815), convinced (472), prescribed (638), came (1,436), sensation (543), dizzy (1,099), my (43,208), gotten (420), asleep (613), head (3,050), name (511), ER (540), began (305)
20th	u (207), sister (32), behavior (13), function (24), ur (49), mindfulness (27), chemical (13), learning (29), dog (31), smell (14), balance (33), techniques (30), panicky (19), diet (30), improve (19), mess (22), monitor (21), traumatic (13), brain (120), blood (129), guy (20), journey (21), docs (22), meditation (47), girlfriend (12), doses (11), positive (103), chat (29), awful (70), reassure (16), most (158), rescue (11), less (60), meditate (11), realize (24), thru (18), bc (15), research (21), doc (46), assured (10), hence (10), kidney (10), urine (10), train (14), multiple (14), mg (37)
40th	Google (48), u (115), water (41), lump (14), ya (14), voice (12), trip (15), free (36), peace (27), Paxil (10), otherwise (13), heat (12), stick (15), listen (31), frustrated (10), pretty (38), memory (12), id (11), drinks (10), med (19), ear (22), bath (12), fatigue (12), therapy (53), area (19), information (14), coping (16)
60th	mindfulness (20), ten (10), group (20), nice (42), peace (21), ended (14), somewhere (12), sucks (12), slowly (20), plus (14), tense (11), exercises (10)
Last	university (13), accommodation (10), useful (10), offer (12), simply (11), drink (26), finding (15), yours (11), group (15), emotions (10), mg (15), certain (14), learned (11), write (14), mri (10), mad (10), happens (25), experience (30)

As time went on, they increasingly took on an emotionally supportive or advice-giving role:

> Hi that's **awful** that your psychiatrist just told you to stop taking them. (20th post)

They were also more likely to suggest remedies to anxiety that were based on a non-medicalisation framework:

> I **listen** to mind calming music too which helps me massively to relax. (40th post)

> Going out is my **coping** mechanism even if I do not feel like it or nervous, or apprehensive. (40th post)

It is interesting to note that for people's 20th posts, two linked keywords were *journey* (which metaphorically conceptualised the poster's experience with anxiety) and *learning* (a verb which indicates the continuous or progressive tense), whereas for people's final posts, the keyword *learned* (past tense) was used to provide a summary of the poster's journey, indicating they felt they had made progress and were unlikely to need the group's continuing support.

> I am still **learning** to **improve** what I use and add in a new technique occasionally as well. (20th post)

> **Learning** what works for you is a very personal **journey** but you sound like you know exactly what I mean (20th post)

> I'm back to my old self again, thank God! It was a rough 3 months for me. I've been going to therapy since January and have **learned** to just accept the anxiety and the symptoms. (final post)

While most posters did not make it to their 60th post (indeed, most did not make it to 10 posts), the analysis indicates an interesting sense of progression for the more established posters, in terms of their changing roles in the forum, offering a different perspective on change over time.

7.5 Conclusion

This chapter explored how change over time can be conceived in multiple ways, and analysts are encouraged to not only think about dividing their corpus into years or decades but consider other aspects, such as the age of the text producer(s), repeated cycles (such as the annual cycle), or the length of time that a contributor has been involved in contributing towards an online forum.

The chapter has also shown how different techniques can be used to compare multiple time periods, including the coefficient of variation (CV), the remainder method of keyness, and the use of equation-based graphs and trendlines. Perhaps an unfortunate aspect of most current corpus software is that it does not easily provide procedures for comparing multiple corpora in order to examine change over time (although Sketch Engine's 'Trends' function is an exception). Therefore, it is often necessary to supplement the corpus tools with other kinds of software, like Excel or R. The importance of going beyond the corpus, to consider different kinds of social and historical context, should not be understated, and we would recommend that corpus analysts who want to consider change over time also spend some time engaging with frameworks like Resigl and Wodak's Discourse Historical Analysis approach (2001) as a means of explaining their findings.

References

Baker, C. (2019). *Obesity Statistics. House of Commons Briefing Paper 3336*. House of Commons. Available at https://researchbriefings.files.parliament.uk/documents/SN03336/SN03336.pdf.
Baker, P. (2017). *American and British English. Divided by a Common Language?* Cambridge University Press.
Collins, L. and Baker, P. (2023). *Language, Discourse and Anxiety*. Cambridge University Press.
Corrigan, D. and Scarlett, M. (2020). *Health Survey (NI): First Results 2018/19*. Northern Ireland Department of Health. www.health-ni.gov.uk/sites/default/files/publications/health/hsni-first-results-18-19_1.pdf.
Leech, G., Hundt, M., Mair, C. and Smith, N. (2009). *Change in Contemporary English: A Grammatical Study*. Cambridge University Press.
National Statistics (2018). *Statistics on Obesity, Physical Activity and Diet*. NHS Digital. https://files.digital.nhs.uk/publication/0/0/obes-phys-acti-diet-eng-2018-rep.pdf.
Rayson, P. (2008). From Key Words to Key Semantic Domains. *International Journal of Corpus Linguistics*, *13*(4), 519–49. https://doi.org/10.1075/ijcl.13.4.06ray.
Reisigl, M. and Wodak, R. (2001). *Discourse and Discrimination: Rhetorics of Racism and Antisemitism*. Routledge.
Scott, M. (2016). *WordSmith Tools* (version 7). Lexical Analysis Software.
Scottish Government (2017). *Obesity Indicators*. Scotland: Official Statistics. Available at www.gov.scot/publications/obesity-indicators-monitoring-progress-prevention-obesity-route-map/.

8 Historical Data

8.1 Introduction

The previous chapter considered change over short periods of time involving health-related corpora that reflected present-day language use. There is a long-standing tradition within corpus linguistics of analysing historical language data (e.g., Taavitsainen et al., 2014). In this chapter we also consider time, yet here we consider language use over longer stretches of time using historical corpora. In dealing with data which is remote in time, more groundwork often needs to be carried out in terms of locating and cleaning texts and forming relevant research questions (as already mentioned in Chapter 3). A detailed consideration of context is also important, in order to provide interpretations and explanations of findings which are informed, for example, by historiography. Accordingly, when looking at such data, we have found that it can be very helpful to include a historian as part of the research team.

In the following sections we will look at two case studies. The first explores an issue – vaccination – that is widely discussed in public discourse, both in the past and in the present day. The second case study – on the topic of sexually transmitted diseases (STDs) – is more exploratory and faced challenges in terms of identifying relevant examples in the corpus. This led to an analysis of collocates, which in turn resulted in the identification of new research questions.

8.2 Anti-vaccination Discourse in Nineteenth-Century England

In Chapter 3 we discussed the rationale and process for the construction of the Victorian Vaccination Discourse corpus (VicVaDis) – a 3.5-million-word collection of anti-vaccination material published in England between 1854 and 1906. During that period (which roughly overlaps with the reign of Queen Victoria), a series of Vaccination Acts made the vaccine against smallpox compulsory for babies at three months of age and imposed penalties on parents who did not comply, including fines and, potentially, imprisonment. Response to the Vaccination Acts included a large-scale organised anti-vaccination movement

8.2 Anti-vaccination Discourse in 19th-Century England

that persisted until a Vaccination Act in 1907 made conscientious objection easier, to the extent that in practice compulsion no longer applied. Contentious as they may have been, the Vaccination Acts marked the beginning of a process which led, thanks to vaccination, to the eventual eradication of smallpox in 1980.

As noted in Chapter 3, in 1853 immunisation against smallpox in England involved the insertion of material from the pustules of people infected with cowpox – a mild disease which had been found to confer protection against the much more dangerous smallpox in humans. Previous work based on document analysis had identified three main concerns about compulsory smallpox vaccination in nineteenth-century England (Durbach, 2005; Fajri Nuwarda et al., 2022). The first concern involved potential dangers to health. This was partly because of some inherent risks involved in vaccination practices at the time, but there were also broader beliefs that vaccination interferes with what might be seen as the purity of the human body. The second concern related to the later practice of propagating the cowpox virus on the skin of calves and sheep – the resultant vaccination was viewed as the insertion of animal products into people, which raised religious objections. The third concern involved civil liberties and the mandatory nature of vaccination; critics objected to the penalties that applied to non-compliant parents, particularly from the poorer sections of society.

The availability of the VicVaDis corpus makes it possible to systematically investigate the manifestations of these different concerns in a collection of pamphlets and other texts that were widely available at the time, as well as to identify further patterns of objections. In turn, these can be compared with what is known about vaccine-hesitant views from other historical periods – particularly the present day.

In the rest of this section, we will report the main findings of an initial analysis of the VicVaDis corpus carried out by Hardaker and co-authors (2024), and complement these findings with further observations we have made by exploring the corpus, which can be freely accessed from the website of the Questioning Vaccination Discourse project (www.lancaster.ac.uk/vaccination-discourse/vicvadis/).

8.2.1 'Vaccination' and 'Compulsory' in the VicVaDis Corpus

Hardaker and co-authors (2024) approached the question of vaccination by looking at how it was represented in Victorian textual material and comparing that to how similar concepts are represented today. They began their exploration of the VicVaDis corpus by focusing on the noun *vaccination*, which is the most frequent lexical word in the corpus, with 31,734 occurrences (9,095.55 per million words). This is, of course, not surprising, given the way in which texts were selected for inclusion in the corpus in the first place. Nonetheless, starting from the most frequent lexical words provides a data-driven rationale for the exploration of the corpus. The collocation tool in the corpus search software AntConc (Anthony, 2022) was used to compute the collocates of *vaccination* within a span of five words to the left and five words to the right of the node word. They then examined the adjective *compulsory*, which is the most frequent open-class collocate of 'vaccination' (log likelihood = 5,583.747; effect size using mutual information = 3.032).

Out of 2,223 occurrences of the collocational pair, a random sample of 500 concordance lines were examined manually for arguments against vaccination. This revealed some patterns that were both characteristic of the historical period represented in the corpus and comparable to anti-vaccination concerns and arguments that still apply today.

In the 1800s, one of the charges that was repeatedly levelled against smallpox vaccination was that it was ineffective. In the following extract, this claim is supported by quantitative data showing that there appears to be no clear or steady decline in the number of infections over time:

> The compulsory vaccination laws came into operation in 1854 and you would naturally expect that there would be a continuous decrease in mortality. What are the facts? In 1858, 1861, 1864 and 1867, the deaths from smallpox were 6,460, 1,320, 7,684 and 2,115 respectively. (Pickering, 1871, in *Vaccination: A Letter in Reply to an Article in the "Leeds Mercury"*)

Hardaker and co-authors (2024) point out a specific parallel with contemporary discussions regarding the effectiveness of the HPV vaccine. HPV protects against a number of cancers and diseases caused by different strains of the human papillomavirus, but in particular it protects against cervical cancer and there is increasing evidence for the effectiveness of HPV vaccination campaigns in reducing cervical cancer rates (Palmer et al., 2024). There is increasing evidence for the effectiveness of HPV vaccination campaigns in reducing cervical cancer rates (Palmer et al., 2024). However, in a 2019 study, it was found that concerns about efficacy and the length of protection were among the top sources of hesitancy in relation to this vaccine (Karaphillakis et al., 2019).

Another objection in the Victorian era was that, as a human-made process, vaccination was unnatural:

> This compulsory Vaccination, which is a wanton outrage upon nature, a stupid blunder of man, betrays also an unaccountable blindness, ignorance, or entire suppression of wrong nor human slaughter, but by the application of the powers of nature to the improvement of mankind. (Halket, 1870, *Compulsory Vaccination!! A Crime against Nature!! An Outrage upon Society!!*)

Similarly, Kata (2012), in a study of anti-vaccination websites, identified among the most common 'tropes' the claim that vaccines should be rejected as unnatural, as compared with immunity acquired via infection or alternative approaches to prevention (see also Fasce et al., 2023).

8.2 Anti-vaccination Discourse in 19th-Century England

A related argument is that disease can be prevented by living hygienically and morally, so that vaccination is unnecessary:

> The only efficient prophylactic against disease, whether smallpox, fever &c, is to be found in enlightened and faithful compliance with the laws of life and health, which these compulsory vaccination laws- by teaching people to trust in vaccination and leading them to believe that they may nourish with impunity the real causes of smallpox- set utterly and daringly at defiance. (Pickering, 1873, *The Antivaccinator and Public Health Journal*)

This is similar to an argument that is sometimes made to refuse or delay HPV vaccination for adolescent girls in particular. As HPV is submitted via sexual contact, it is sometimes (mistakenly) suggested that infection can be avoided by limiting the number of (usually women's) sexual partners. In this way, vaccination is presented as necessary only for people with supposedly 'risky' sexual habits (Hendry et al., 2013; Semino et al., 2023). More generally, the idea that 'hygienic' lifestyles are a preferable alternative to vaccination has consistently been identified in anti-vaccination arguments in studies drawing from online twenty-first-century data (Fasce et al., 2023, Kata, 2012).

Hardaker and co-authors also identify a variety of manifestations of the view that mandatory vaccinations are incompatible with civil liberties by examining a subset of concordance lines that include the word sequence *compulsory vaccination is*. Examples of what follows this word sequence include:

- 'a great infringement on that freedom which every man has a right to enjoy';
- 'a disgrace to our jurisprudence, and a shameful intrusion upon the rights of personal liberty';
- 'the largest infringement of that freedom ever yet exercised';
- 'almost as disgusting as the forced creed practised by the Inquisition in mediaeval times';
- 'therefore a tyranny that everyone should strenuously resist';
- 'a system of tyranny and torture; I use the word advisedly'; and
- 'to surrender the cardinal principle of civil and religious liberty, and to establish a precedent for the exercise of any form of tyranny' (Hardaker et al., 2024: 170).

An examination of these concordance lines also reveals how highly emotional extended metaphors were used to highlight the consequences of compulsory vaccination for citizens' freedoms:

> A wider, and deeper, and subtler *Social* Evil than universal Compulsory Vaccination is scarcely conceivable; ... Politically, *Compulsory Vaccination* is an innermost stab of Liberty which piercing its heart, will find its courage and licaven-bom [*heaven-born*] principles and convictions in other directions an easy

prey. State medicine can do what it Ukes [*likes*] with us, if we once let it do this. (London Society for the Abolition of Compulsory Vaccination (1879), *The Vaccination Inquirer and Health Review: The Organ of the London Society*)

Hardaker and co-authors (2024) point out that in this extract, the author of a letter to the president and members of the International Congress on Compulsory Vaccination personifies 'Liberty' as the victim of physical aggression to support the 'slippery slope' argument that accepting compulsory vaccination will inevitably lead to further and ever more pernicious erosions of personal liberties.

At the time of this writing, no vaccinations are mandatory in England and the United Kingdom more broadly. However, similar concerns about the violation of fundamental freedoms as well as the creation of inequalities were expressed during the COVID-19 pandemic at the prospect of vaccination being compulsory for people employed in certain sectors (notably health and social care) and for the purposes of international travel (Jecker, 2022).

8.2.2 Keywords in the VicVaDis Corpus

Hardaker and co-authors (2024) also utilised the AntConc software to identify the keywords – or statistically 'overused' words – in the VicVaDis corpus (see Chapter 3). This required the creation of a reference corpus from the same variety of English and historical periods. The Corpus of Late Modern English Texts v.3.1 (CLMET3.1), compiled by De Smet and colleagues (2015; http://fedora.clarin-d.uni-saarland.de/clmet/clmet.html), was identified as a suitable source of data. It contains texts produced in the period 1790 to 1920, classified by genre, for a total of 34 million words. Hardaker and colleagues extracted all texts classified under the genre labels 'treatise' and 'letters' and written between 1850 and 1907, to match as closely as possible the inclusion criteria for the VicVaDis corpus. The result was a reference corpus, VicRef, which contains 1,947,789 tokens of comparable dates and genres as the VicVaDis corpus.

Hardaker and colleagues reported the top-25 keywords (Table 8.1; reproduced from Hardaker et al., 2024: 171) and focus on four specific lexical items than can potentially refer both to what is prevented by vaccination (i.e., smallpox) and to what is allegedly caused by vaccination (i.e., a variety of side effects or vaccine harms): *death, deaths, disease*, and *diseases*. For the purposes of the present chapter, we also consider the keyword *cases*. These five keywords appear in bold in Table 8.1.

Out of 7,207 occurrences of *death/deaths*, 861 (11.9 per cent) were found to involve deaths attributed to smallpox itself (e.g., 'deaths by smallpox' or 'death after smallpox'), while 340 (4.7 per cent) were found to involve deaths attributed to vaccination (e.g., 'deaths from vaccination' and 'deaths due to vaccination'). The latter included cases where it was claimed that the

Table 8.1 Top 25 keywords from VicVaDis when compared with VicRef, ordered by keyness (log likelihood)

Rank	Type	Raw frequency: VicVaDis	Raw frequency: VicRef	Normalised frequency per million words: VicVaDis	Normalised frequency per million words: VicRef	Keyness (likelihood)	Keyness (effect)
1	vaccination	31,734	4	9,095.55	2.005	28,736.667	0.018
2	smallpox	21,874	4	6,269.492	2.005	19,765.969	0.012
3	vaccinated	8,876	3	2,544.025	1.504	7,988.536	0.005
4	**disease**	**8,592**	**116**	**2,462.626**	**58.142**	**6,780.952**	**0.005**
5	dr	11,186	636	3,206.114	318.781	6,459.756	0.006
6	medical	7,793	64	2,233.618	32.079	6,441.045	0.004
7	jenner	5,345	0	1,531.976	0	4,837.453	0.003
8	cowpox	4,687	0	1,343.381	0	4,241.613	0.003
9	mr	9,608	1,140	2,753.83	571.399	3,731.588	0.005
10	lymph	3,586	5	1,027.814	2.506	3,179.169	0.002
11	was	29,005	8,671	8,313.368	4,346.144	3,141.183	0.016
12	vaccine	3,517	8	1,008.037	4.01	3,085.139	0.002
13	inoculation	3,416	3	979.089	1.504	3,048.773	0.002
14	**deaths**	**3,441**	**28**	**986.254**	**14.034**	**2,844.497**	**0.002**
15	mortality	3,373	34	966.764	17.042	2,739.78	0.002
16	compulsory	2,989	14	856.703	7.017	2,554.487	0.002
17	epidemic	2,867	9	821.735	4.511	2,490.431	0.002
18	years	7,150	997	2,049.322	499.724	2,430.964	0.004
19	**diseases**	**3,059**	**40**	**876.766**	**20.049**	**2,421.166**	**0.002**
20	unvaccinated	2,184	0	625.975	0	1,975.893	0.001
21	**cases**	**6,258**	**962**	**1,793.658**	**482.181**	**1,940.183**	**0.004**
22	cannot	2,116	0	606.485	0	1,914.357	0.001
23	london	4,198	443	1,203.224	222.044	1,770.514	0.002
24	hospital	2,276	36	652.344	18.044	1,760.796	0.001
25	**death**	**3,739**	**335**	**1,071.666**	**167.911**	**1,744.884**	**0.002**

extent of deaths caused by vaccination was being covered up by not mentioning vaccination in death certificates:

> In October 1876 an official inquiry was made concerning the illnesses through vaccination of sixteen children in the Misterton district of the Gainsborough Union, of which six proved fatal, but no mention was made of vaccination in any of the **death** certificates. Of the four deaths at Norwich, the subject also of an official inquiry in 1882, only one was certified as being due to vaccination. It appeared that nine children were vaccinated in June by Dr. Guy, the public vaccinator; of these four were dead of erysipelas within three weeks of the operation, and five were seriously ill from constitutional disease. (Tebb, 1889, *What Is the Truth about Vaccination?*)

Hardaker and colleagues point out that this charge of cover-up is still made today in arguments against vaccination. For example, during the COVID-19 pandemic, it was found that many vaccine-hesitant individuals believed that the official figures for deaths caused by COVID-19 were inflated and that the actual number of deaths caused by the vaccines was concealed (Jones et al., 2023).

The keywords *disease/diseases* occur 12,078 times in the corpus and can be used to refer to smallpox itself or to diseases that are allegedly caused by the vaccine. In the former cases, occurrences of *disease/diseases* tend to be part of claims about the ineffectiveness of the vaccine:

> There appears to be no positive security against the **disease**, either by vaccination or by smallpox inoculation, and I have seen several cases where the patients have caught smallpox twice, and have each time been very severely marked; and in two instances have died of the second attack of smallpox. (Pearce, 1868, *Vaccination: Its Tested Effects on Health, Mortality, and Population – An Essay*)

As previously mentioned, such arguments are also made against current vaccines, especially in cases where vaccines offer relatively low levels of protection against disease, as in the case of vaccines against the flu and COVID-19.

In contrast, in cases such as the following extract, the noun *diseases* occurs as part of allegations that the vaccine does more harm than smallpox itself:

> For every child that dies from smallpox, forty die from **diseases** induced by Vaccination. (LSACV, 1879, *The Vaccination Inquirer and Health Review: The Organ of the London Society*)

The nineteenth-century version of the smallpox vaccine involved the injection of bodily fluids containing live cowpox virus into babies' arms. It thus carried more dangers of a variety of side effects, some of them serious. In addition, the kind of anti-vaccination material that was included in the VicVaDis corpus blamed vaccination for a very wide variety of harmful consequences.

To investigate such allegations, in this chapter we additionally consider the keyword *cases*, which has 6,258 occurrences in the corpus (1,940.183 per million

8.2 Anti-vaccination Discourse in 19th-Century England

words). Where the noun *cases* is not followed by references to smallpox itself (e.g., 'cases of smallpox'), it tends to be followed by references to problems, symptoms, or diseases that are presented as the consequence of vaccination. The most frequently mentioned is the skin infection erysipelas:

> The official report of the Imperial Foundling hospital at St. Petersburg for the year 1864, the cases of erysipelas after vaccination are given as 156, of whom 2 died. (Wilkinson et al., 1879, *Vaccination Tracts*)

Other references to harms presented as being caused by vaccination in the concordance lines for *cases* include *cancer, eczema, erythema, gangrenous eruption, leprosy, lupus, prurigo, septic poisoning, syphilisation, syphilitic infection*, and *tetanus*.

We do not have the space to discuss the medical and scientific basis for each of these claims. We can, however, point out that the list of harms attributed to vaccination includes a lot of variation in terms of both plausibility and seriousness. Even the modern version of the smallpox vaccine can cause or exacerbate skin problems such as eczema (Belongia and Naleway, 2003). Conversely, the list of harms also includes at least some cases that could be described in contemporary terms as mis- or disinformation. The most obvious is cancer:

> In my individual experience a number of **cases of** cancer and sarcoma seem to have been directly traceable to vaccination as a cause. (Furnival, 1906, *Professional Opinion Adverse to Vaccination*)

During the writing of this book, similarly unsubstantiated allegations were made on social media that the cancer diagnosis revealed in March 2024 by the Princess of Wales was a result of the COVID-19 vaccines.

As Hardaker and colleagues put it,

> perhaps the most intriguing aspect of VicVaDis is that it demonstrates with remarkable clarity that the modern fears around new vaccines, such as those developed in light of COVID-19, are in fact not modern at all. Each new vaccine – smallpox, HPV, MMR, COVID-19 – may have its unique components and concerns, but the genesis of the fears themselves appears to remain relatively stable over the centuries. This data suggests that we continue to struggle with how best to assess the risks posed by the diseases themselves versus those posed by the vaccines, how to protect our children when we are required to make decisions on their behalf that have potentially severe or even fatal outcomes, how to protect our rights to make those decisions in the face of contradictory advice or mandates, where and how to draw causative links in a febrile medical arena clouded with doubts and loudly competing voices, and so forth. (Hardaker et al., 2024: 172)

The availability and exploitation of historical corpora such as VicVaDis can make an important contribution to the comparative study of discourse and social phenomena across times and cultures.

8.3 Representations around Sexually Transmitted Diseases in Early English Books Online

In this section we outline a study which provides insight into how data can help us research while challenging analysts to both revise their research questions and improve the data they use. The study also shows how a shift in the contemporary context in which work is conducted may create a relevance for a research project that was not the intended goal of the project but was, nonetheless, its outcome.

The study was part of a long-standing research programme using corpus data from the early modern period to explore marginalised identities in seventeenth-century English writing. The data in question was Early English Books Online (EEBO), a digitised collection of more than 146,000 printed works in English produced largely before 1700. This database had originally been made available as scanned images which granted researchers access to these texts without the need for expensive field trips to libraries. While these scans were of limited use to corpus linguists – they could not be searched using corpus software – they did at least allow key works to be consulted at scale, with work such as McEnery (2006) using EEBO, to explore the use of 'bad language' in Early Modern English. The scans were often derived from poor-quality texts. Even so, optical character recognition (OCR) scanning of these texts made it possible for users to search for a word in order to determine which pages from which texts might be of interest. While the results were prone to a high degree of error, the search function was still helpful. The process of improving the utility of the data began in 1999 when a group called the Text Creation Partnership (TCP) was formed, consisting of University of Michigan Library, Bodleian Libraries at the University of Oxford, ProQuest, and the Council on Library and Information Resources. The TCP worked to produce high-fidelity, machine-readable, textual transcriptions of the documents in EEBO. The resulting data *was* suitable for corpus analysis. In the work reported here, EEBO version 3 was used, providing just under a billion words of data for the seventeenth century. A billion words would, in the recent past, have presented its own challenges to standard corpus search packages, exceeding by far the limits of those software packages to search the data. However, the work on EEBO reported here used CQPweb (Hardie, 2012), which allows the rapid search and analysis of multi-billion-word corpora.

While the EEBO data still presented challenges, these were challenges linguists always had to face when working with data from this period – for example, limited metadata and variant spellings which made it difficult to search for all the occurrences of a specific word. Nonetheless, EEBO TCP opened up new avenues of possibility for corpus linguists, and in the programme of work described here, a corpus linguist and a historian worked

8.3 Representations around Sexually Transmitted Diseases   127

together to carry on in the spirit of the work of McEnery (2006) to look at the representation of marginalised groups such as the poor (McEnery and Baker, 2019) and prostitutes (McEnery and Baker, 2017).

In pursuing their research on marginalised groups in the early modern period, the researchers used methods from corpus linguistics; where appropriate, these were supplemented with other methods, notably geographical information systems, to explore the locations where marginalised groups resided (Baker et al., 2019). The analysis blended the close reading and critical archive research of a historian with insights provided by linguists and corpus data.

The study summarised here began with a research question in a similar vein to those discussed previously – the researchers wanted to look at the representation of people with STDs in the seventeenth century (McEnery and Baker, 2022). While EEBO addressed the issue of access to a sufficient volume of data, availability was only the first challenge. While earlier work had proved possible with the data, when the researchers sought to explore the representation of people with STDs in EEBO, they encountered a substantial problem – one of the primary terms for referring to STDs, *pox*, was also a very frequent swear word of the time. It was also a very frequent word – there were 9,960 examples of *pox* in the section of the corpus covering the seventeenth century. With so many occurrences, reading all of the concordance lines to distinguish mentions of STDs from the use of the term as a curse or an insult would have been prohibitively time-consuming. An alternative approach would be to work with a sample of the data, which would have allowed the analysts to broadly characterise the usage of the word. As a way of trying to down-sample the data in a principled way, the analysts turned to collocation (see Chapter 1).[1] This approach proved partly helpful. Some collocates clearly related to cursing, such as *rogue*, which collocated with *pox* 30 times in the corpus and never referred to STDs, being used instead as a curse (e.g., in sentences such as 'A pox on you for a rogue').[2]

However, the collocates also revealed a further problem, along with presenting two opportunities. The problem related to those examples of *pox* which clearly related to disease. As the word refers to a symptom of disease, a pustule and its consequent scarring of the skin, it is quite vague as a term. On examining the examples of *pox* clearly related to disease, the researchers could see that only in a subset of cases could they be sure of the nature of the disease causing the pock marks. Collocates such as *venerous*, occurring 12 times, always in the fixed expression *venerous pox*, clearly relate to what would now be called

---

[1] In the examples cited here, we used the log ratio statistic to identify collocates, using a span of five words to the left and right as our collocation window and a minimum of five co-occurrences of the word searched for and a specific collocate to filter out low-frequency cases.
[2] From *Cambridge Jests, or, Witty Alarums for Melancholy Spirit* by an anonymous author under the pseudonym 'Lover of ha, ha, he', published in 1674 by Samuel Lowndes.

syphilis. Yet when the word collocates with other STDs, such as *gonorrhoea*, it is not necessarily the case that *pox* is indicating syphilis. In some cases it probably does as it is linked to other venereal diseases (e.g., 'cures the greatest Pox, Gonorrhea's, Cankers, and all Venereal Diseases').[3] However, the word may also appear in a list of diseases and be ambiguous, as in 'the Gonorrhea, Pox, Gout, Leprosy, and other such like Diseases perfectly cured'.[4] That ambiguity is made apparent when we consider other collocates which indicate various diseases collocating with *pox* that are also linked to pock marks, notably *small* producing *small pox* (mentioned 2,001 times in the seventeenth-century data).

Yet one type of collocate always denoted an STD and was of interest from the point of view of discourse analysis – nationality terms (e.g., *French pox*). Through such examples, the agency of the infection was, in part, ascribed to foreigners. This offered an opportunity, resulting in the analysts reconsidering their research question. Rather than focusing on the construction of those afflicted with the disease, they decided to focus on the agency for the introduction of the disease. This was both tractable as a research question and somewhat contested in the literature. The insight gained from that collocation allowed the exploration of a new, and fruitful, angle on STDs in discourse in seventeenth-century England.

The second opportunity that the collocation analysis provided related to the close reading that was carried out to support the interpretation of collocates. Through looking at the examples and checking the metadata to ascertain the date of the example and the name of the text in which it was written, an impression was formed that certain collocates of *pox* increased over time, but they also increasingly appeared in certain types of texts as the century progressed. As the texts were marked with a date of publication, it was easy to explore how a term such as *French pox* was dispersed over time. There were 1,181 such examples in the seventeenth century, and when the researchers looked at the relative frequency of the term in the decades across that century, it was found that the peak of mention for the term occurred in the 1650s (1.78 examples per million words), with a later peak in the 1690s (1 example per million words). While there was no reliable metadata that enabled an examination of distribution of the terms by genre of text, scattered, compelling evidence was found that suggested a link between time and genre relating to *pox*. For example, when exploring the texts in which *pox* and *rogue* collocated, all but two were clearly plays.

To explore the link between the construction of the disease in terms of nationality on the one hand, and genre of text on the other, it was decided to

---

[3] From *Choice and Experimented Receipts in Physick and Chirurgery* by Sir Kenelm Digby, published in 1675 by Andrew Clark.
[4] From *The Marrow of Chymical Physick* by William Thrasher, published in 1679 by Peter Parke.

8.3 Representations around Sexually Transmitted Diseases 129

produce a genre classification of all the texts in the EEBO v.3 corpus. The process of doing that is described in McEnery and Baker (2022), but in brief the authors used the titles of the works in question, supported by a limited amount of close reading, to first develop a genre classification of the texts in the corpus and then assign texts to that classification. The classification itself was composed of five major genres (Literary, Religious, Administrative, Instructional, and Informational), which were further divided and subdivided to produce a total of 25 sub-genres and 80 sub-sub-genres. The classification was further developed and used in a subsequent project focused on the creation of a dictionary of Shakespeare's language (see Culpeper et al., 2023; Murphy, 2019). While painstaking, the genre classification task enabled the exploration of the link between nationality, STDs, and genre.

The analysis found that while there was a wide range of nationalities associated with the pox, French people were most frequently linked to it. This gave plausibility to claims in the literature that proximity was a driver in the naming of such diseases – English writers blamed a local rival power. Three main terms were used for this, in descending order of frequency: *French pox*, *French disease*, and *morbus gallicus*. By normalising the frequency of mentions to per million words, the terms were seen to peak in use in the 1650s and 1660s, fall, and then rise in frequency again in the 1690s. However, there was also an elevated mention of *Naples* with reference to the pox, as English writers did, on occasion, mention the possibility that it was in fact Naples that was the source of the disease and more specifically soldiers of the army of Charles VIII who had marched on and captured Naples. However, as Charles was a French king at the head of a French army, this also, indirectly, pinned the blame on France. So while the *Neapolitan pox* may have been linked to Naples, more broadly it was still linked to France in wider discourse.

The genre analysis of the corpus corroborated the hypothesis that the discussion of the geographical origins of STDs varied by genre and through time. The main finding of the genre analysis was that, as the century proceeded, the discussion of French pox rose substantially in one genre: medical writing. By 1690, the number of mentions of French pox (and associated variations) had grown. From the 1630s onwards, it occurred most often in medical texts, and by the 1690s, the term was barely used in any other genre. Prior to the 1630s, there was a peak of mentions of syphilis in the genre labelled as treatise (a form of formal writing systematically investigating a particular subject), in which French pox was linked to a range of topics, including anti-Catholicism and the discussion of far-off places. Peaks in this period of texts from the history genre tend to discuss the possible geographical origins of the disease.

After a series of initial difficulties working with the data, the analysts were able to both usefully refocus their initial research question and enrich the data to discover new insights into the framing of discussions of disease in terms of blame and agency. In this case, both of those converge on one party – the French. However, as the century proceeds, we see the discourse around the disease shifting markedly towards medicalisation. That medicalisation is apparent in the pattern of collocation surrounding the phrase *French pox* – if the top-10 collocates of this word are considered in the medical writing in the corpus, it is seen that they relate to other diseases (*scurvy, dropsy, leprosy, gout, diseases*), medical treatments (*dose, cures, cured, cure*), and the process of infection (*infected*). As the discussion of *French pox* rises in this genre, by association this medicalised framing of it also rises. Importantly, if the collocates across the whole corpus are examined, it is seen that while collocates relating to other diseases are typical of general usage, the mention of supposed cures (*cinnabar, guajacum, quick silver*), moral judgements (*evil*), and naming strategies (*called, Naples*) are present in general English but not medical discourse. The rise of a medicalised discourse around French pox, therefore, is also marked by a move away from a culture of blaming, moralising, and bogus cures.

At this point it appeared that the work on this data was complete. However, in the process of submitting the work for publication, an event occurred that impacted on the publication itself. The work was submitted for publication in late 2019, just before the COVID-19 pandemic struck. Early in the COVID-19 pandemic, a process began of linking the disease, and its variants, to specific geographies, just as had happened with syphilis centuries before. The initial set of reviews for the paper asked that this be acknowledged, which was done. After resubmission, the public debate around COVID-19 had moved on, and the practice of linking COVID variants to the places in which they were detected had been much reduced, to avoid stigmatising national groups. When the paper returned from its second review, the reviewer noted this and asked that the researchers remove the reference to COVID-19 from the paper. The request was discussed with the editor, and ultimately the researchers decided to leave the reference in, as the paper was precisely about how geography and disease can combine to stigmatise. COVID-19, appearing in the publication process when it did, showed just how little had changed in terms of disease-naming practices, while also being illustrative of how naming practices can be just as sensitive and harmful today as they were four centuries ago.

8.4 Conclusion

Historical data can be much more difficult to collect, particularly if one wants to ensure a fully representative corpus. Poor OCR transfers or natural spelling variation can make it especially difficult to carry out lexicographic analysis based on word frequencies in such a context. Tools like VARD (Baron and Rayson, 2008) can help introduce a degree of systematic standardisation into historical corpus data. There is also the possibility that artificial intelligence

8.4 Conclusion

software will be able to further improve on poorly scanned historical data, though that promise lies in the future at the time of this writing.

As the two case studies have shown, one aspect of historical corpus research on health-related topics is that the findings can sometimes help shed new light on more contemporary topics, showing how discourses can sometimes remain remarkably entrenched or are able to resurface, given similar conditions. However, there is a danger when analysing historical corpora in assuming that the attitudes and language use of the past are the same as the present. Unlike the corpora examined in the previous chapter, we do not have direct experience in the time period that these corpus texts were written in, and thus we should not impose our own values on the authors of historical texts. Context is key – it is notable how the first case study in this chapter cites large chunks of texts in order to better make sense of the use of a keyword, whereas in the second case study it was necessary to classify the genres of texts before they could be analysed. Additionally, we often need to go beyond the texts themselves, to account more holistically for the time period that they were produced in, which is one of the reasons why it can be useful to work with a historian in this challenging but rewarding form of health linguistics.

References

Anthony, L. (2022). AntConc (Version 4.2.0) [Computer Software]. Tokyo: Waseda University. Available from www.laurenceanthony.net/software.

Baker, H., Gregory, I., Hartmann, D. and McEnery, T. (2019). Applying Geographical Information Systems to Researching Historical Corpora: Seventeenth Century Prostitution. In V. Wiegand and M. Mahlberg (eds.), *Corpus Linguistics, Context and Culture* (pp. 109–36). De Gruyter.

Baron, A. and Rayson, P. (2008). VARD 2: A Tool for Dealing with Spelling Variation in Historical Corpora. *Proceedings of the Postgraduate Conference in Corpus Linguistics*, Aston University, Birmingham, UK, 22 May 2008.

Belongia, E. A. and Naleway, A. L. (2003). Smallpox Vaccine: The Good, the Bad, and the Ugly. *Clinical Medicine and Research*, *1*(2), 87–92. https://doi.org/10.3121/cmr.1.2.87.

Culpeper, J., Hardie, A. and Demmen, J. (2023). *The Arden Encyclopaedia of Shakespeare's Language*. Bloomsbury.

Durbach, N. (2005). *Bodily Matters. The Anti-vaccination Movement in England, 1853–1907*. Duke University Press.

Fajri Nuwarda, R., Ramzan, I., Weekes, L. and Kayser, V. (2022). Vaccine Hesitancy: Contemporary Issues and Historical Background. *Vaccines*, *10*(10), 1595. https://doi.org/10.3390/vaccines10101595.

Fasce, A., Schmid, P., Holford, D. L., Bates, L., Gurevych, I. and Lewandowsky, S. (2023). A Taxonomy of Anti-vaccination Arguments from a Systematic Literature Review and Text Modelling. *Nature Human Behaviour*, *7*(9), 1462–80. https://doi.org/10.1038/s41562-023-01644-3.

Hardaker, C., Deignan, A., Semino, E., Coltman-Patel, T., Dance, W., Demjén, Z., Sanderson, C. and Gatherer, D. (2024). The Victorian Anti-Vaccination Discourse Corpus (VicVaDis): Construction and Exploration. *Digital Scholarship in the Humanities*, *39*, 162–74. https://doi.org/10.1093/llc/fqad075.

Hardie, A. (2012). CQPweb – Combining Power, Flexibility and Usability in a Corpus Analysis Tool. *International Journal of Corpus Linguistics*, *17*(3), 380–409. https://doi.org/10.1075/ijcl.17.3.04har.

Hendry, M., Lewis, R., Clements, A., Damery, S. and Wilkinson C. (2013). 'HPV? Never Heard of It!': A Systematic Review of Girls' and Parents' Information Needs, Views and Preferences about Human Papillomavirus Vaccination. *Vaccine*, *25*(45), 5152–67. https://doi.org/10.1016/j.vaccine.2013.08.091.

Jecker, N. S. (2022). Vaccine Passports and Health Disparities: A Perilous Journey. *Journal of Medical Ethics*, *48*, 957–60. https://doi.org/10.1136/medethics-2021-107491.

Jones, L., Bonfield, S., Farrell, J. and Weston, D. (2023). Understanding the Public's Attitudes towards COVID-19 Vaccinations in Nottinghamshire, United Kingdon: Qualitative Social Media Analysis. *Journal of Medical Internet Research*, *25*. https://doi.org/10.2196/38404.

Karaphillakis, E., Simas, C., Jarrett, C., Verger, P., Peretti-Watel, P. and Dib, F. (2019). HPV Vaccination in a Context of Mistrust and Uncertainty: A Systematic Literature Review of Determinants of HPV Vaccine Hesitancy in Europe. *Human Vaccines Immunotherapeutics*, *15*(7–8), 1615–27. https://doi.org/10.1080/21645515.2018.1564436.

Kata, A. (2012). Anti-vaccine Activists, Web 2.0, and the Postmodern Paradigm – An Overview of Tactics and Tropes Used Online by the Anti-vaccination Movement. *Vaccine*, *30*(25), 3778–89. https://doi.org/10.1016/j.vaccine.2011.11.112.

McEnery, T. (2006). *Swearing in English: Bad Language, Purity and Power 1586 to the Present*. Routledge.

McEnery, T. and Baker, H. (2017). *Corpus Linguistics and 17th Century Prostitution*. Bloomsbury.

(2019). Language Surrounding Poverty in Early Modern England: A Corpus Based Investigation of How People Living in the Seventeenth Century Perceived the Criminalized Poor. In C. Suhr, T. Nevalainen and I. Taavitsainen (eds.), *From Data to Evidence in English Language Research* (pp. 225–57). Brill.

(2022). A Geography of Names: A Genre Analysis of Nationality-Driven Names for Venereal Disease in the Seventeenth Century. In T. Hiltunen and I. Taavitsainen (eds.), *Corpus Pragmatic Studies on the History of Medical Discourse* (pp. 23–48). John Benjamins.

Murphy, S. (2019). Shakespeare and His Contemporaries: Designing a Genre Classification Scheme for Early English Books Online 1560–1640. *ICAME Journal*, *43*(1), 59–82. https://doi.org/10.2478/icame-2019-0003.

Palmer, T. J., Kavanagh, K., Cuschieri, K., Cameron, R., Graham, C., Wilson, A. and Roy, K. (2024). Invasive Cervical Cancer Incidence Following Bivalent Human Papillomavirus Vaccination: A Population-Based Observational Study of Age at Immunization, Dose, and Deprivation. *JNCI: Journal of the National Cancer Institute*, *116*(6), 857–65. https://doi.org/10.1093/jnci/djad263.

Semino, E., Coltman-Patel, T., Dance, W., Deignan, A., Demjén, Z., Hardaker, C. and Mackey, A. (2023). Narratives, Information and Manifestations of Resistance to Persuasion in Online Discussions of HPV Vaccination. *Health Communication*, *39* (10), 2123–34. https://doi.org/10.1080/10410236.2023.2257428.

Taavitsainen, I., Hiltunen, T., Lehto, A., Marttila, V., Pahta, P., Ratia, M., Suhr, C. and Tyrkkö, J. (2014). Late Modern English Medical Texts 1700–1800: A Corpus for Analysing Eighteenth-Century Medical English. *ICAME Journal*, *38*(1), 137–53. https://doi.org/10.2478/icame-2014-0007.

9 Representing the Experience of Illness

9.1 Introduction

This chapter considers how the experience of illness is represented discursively, focusing on two contexts: anxiety and cancer. Language can be used to represent a single health condition in a range of ways, which is likely to impact the actions that people take in relation to that health condition, with consequences for their well-being. A corpus linguistic approach, using a large quantity of texts, is aptly suited for identifying the different representations or discourses around a health condition, showing the language patterns associated with each of them, and their frequencies of occurrence.

We will first consider a more automatic way of identifying linguistic patterns around a health condition (anxiety), using a tool which identifies the grammatical relationships between a word and its collocates. Although we were not looking for specific forms of language, a common feature we found involved characterisations of anxiety through metaphors. In Section 9.3 we move on to an approach that is based on trying to use corpus techniques to actively identity metaphors.

9.2 Representing Anxiety

This section describes how representations of anxiety were analysed in a 21-million-word corpus of forum posts on the topic of anxiety (described in more detail in Collins and Baker, 2023; see also Sections 5.2 and 7.3 in this book). The forum posts were saved in a single text file, then uploaded into Sketch Engine, an online corpus analysis tool which has several functions that are helpful in terms of identifying patterns in language use. For this study the focus was on the word *anxiety*, which was the twenty-fifth most frequent word in the corpus, occurring 146,874 times. It was the most frequent lexical (open-class) word (with the top 24 words all coming from closed-class categories such as articles like *the* and prepositions like *of*). The noun *anxiety* was also the top keyword when the corpus was compared against the English Web 2020 Corpus (consisting of 38 billion words of internet English collected between 2019 and

2021). However, for a more complete analysis, the researchers could have considered the related adjectival form *anxious* (which occurred 18,217 times). The adjectival form *anxious* suggests a state or feeling which might be temporary, and tends not to reference a medical condition, whereas the related noun form *anxiety* tends to suggest that something is more substantial than a feeling and is a term more widely used in medical discourse. It is notable that the noun form is more than eight times as frequent as the adjectival form in this forum.

Other forms, such as the adverb form *anxiously* or misspellings (e.g., *anxiaty*), were much less frequent (23 and 62 times, respectively) but might have been worth considering to account for every single case. For the purposes of this study, however, only the noun *anxiety* was considered.

9.2.1 Anxiety and Related Terms

Sketch Engine contains a function called Thesaurus, which is based on the theory of distributional semantics to identify synonyms. Thus, words that have similar meanings will share similar collocates. Entering *anxiety* into the Thesaurus produced a list of lexical items, in order of their proportion of shared collocates with *anxiety*. Sketch Engine has a large number of general reference corpora that can be useful to get an idea of how linguistic items typically behave. As such, the analysis began with an examination of *anxiety* in the English Web 2020 Corpus, which contains around a billion words of general English collected from the internet. In this corpus, the 10 words which had the most similar collocates to *anxiety* were *depression, worry, fear, emotion, stress, anger, confusion, frustration, grief,* and *illness*. Intuitively, this makes sense – anxiety is treated in similar ways as negative feelings or mental health conditions – and some of the words on this list (particularly *worry* and *fear*) are similar to *anxiety* and could be subjected to more detailed analyses themselves.

Having obtained an idea of the kind of words that are closest to anxiety in general English, it is now worth focussing in on how it is used in the corpus of forum posts. Here, the top-10 most similar items were *symptom, thing, feeling, attack, I, fear, pain, thought, time,* and *problem*. These words are somewhat different and perhaps less obvious candidates, compared to those elicited through the general corpus, and accordingly they indicate that people with anxiety might have different understandings of their condition. It is interesting, for example, that the word *thing* has similar collocates to *anxiety* in the forum, and concordance analyses found that about 10 per cent of uses of *thing* refer anaphorically to anxiety. For example,

> Anxiety is an awful thing and a vicious circle.

The word *thing* is somewhat vague and general, in addition to being typical of informal ways of communicating. As we will see, there are other ways of conceptualising anxiety, which link to a range of discourses or ways of seeing the world. Therefore, in order to focus more on the collocates of *anxiety* itself, the Word Sketch tool in Sketch Engine was employed. This essentially identifies collocates of *anxiety* and then groups them into grammatical categories. Figure 9.1 shows a (partial) screenshot of a Word Sketch of the word *anxiety*.

The Word Sketch contains several lists of words that collocate with *anxiety*, arranged in order of their collocational strength (with collocational scores hidden as the default), so the numbers in the table relate to the number of times a word collocates with the word *anxiety*. The first column shows nouns that are modified by the word *anxiety*, indicating noun phrases like *anxiety disorder*, *anxiety attack*, and *anxiety symptoms*. The second column shows words (usually adjectives) which modify *anxiety* (e.g., *severe anxiety*). The third column shows adjectives which occur after 'anxiety is'. Due to mistagging, there are sometimes cases that appear in the wrong column (e.g., the word *most* should not be in the adjective predicates list). Finally, the fourth and fifth columns show verbs which collocate with *anxiety*, in the object or subject position, respectively. The fourth column indicates actions which are done to or acted upon anxiety (e.g., *makes my anxiety*), whereas the fifth column shows actions where anxiety is the doer (e.g., *anxiety takes*). The Word Sketch also contains additional columns under these ones (not shown in the figure) which denote further grammatical relationships such as 'anxiety + and/or' or 'pronominal possessors of anxiety'.

This method of grouping collocates into grammatical categories can be helpful for analysts, as it enables them to spot words with similar meanings or functions more easily than a simple list of collocates. In order to identify the various ways that anxiety is represented, it is still necessary for humans to spend time analysing Word Sketch, exploring hypotheses about the ways that collocates position anxiety, through the examination of relevant concordance lines.

For example, in the third column, we can see a number of similar kinds of adjectives that are used to modify *anxiety*: *bad, horrible, awful, hard, severe, terrible*. Taken together, these words would suggest a discourse prosody (Stubbs, 2001) which represents anxiety extremely negatively. Words in other columns also contribute towards this negative depiction (e.g., *severe* and *bad* also appear in the second column), while words like *sufferers* and *problems* in the first column contribute towards the same kind of picture. The word *attack*, in the first column, could also be interpreted as contributing to a negative representation of anxiety.

However, another set of words in the first column seem to represent anxiety somewhat differently: *disorder, symptoms, meds, medication* appear to function in a way which represents anxiety as a medical condition. It is most likely the case that the two representations (anxiety as bad, anxiety as a medical condition) are not incompatible. It is not surprising to see a medical condition

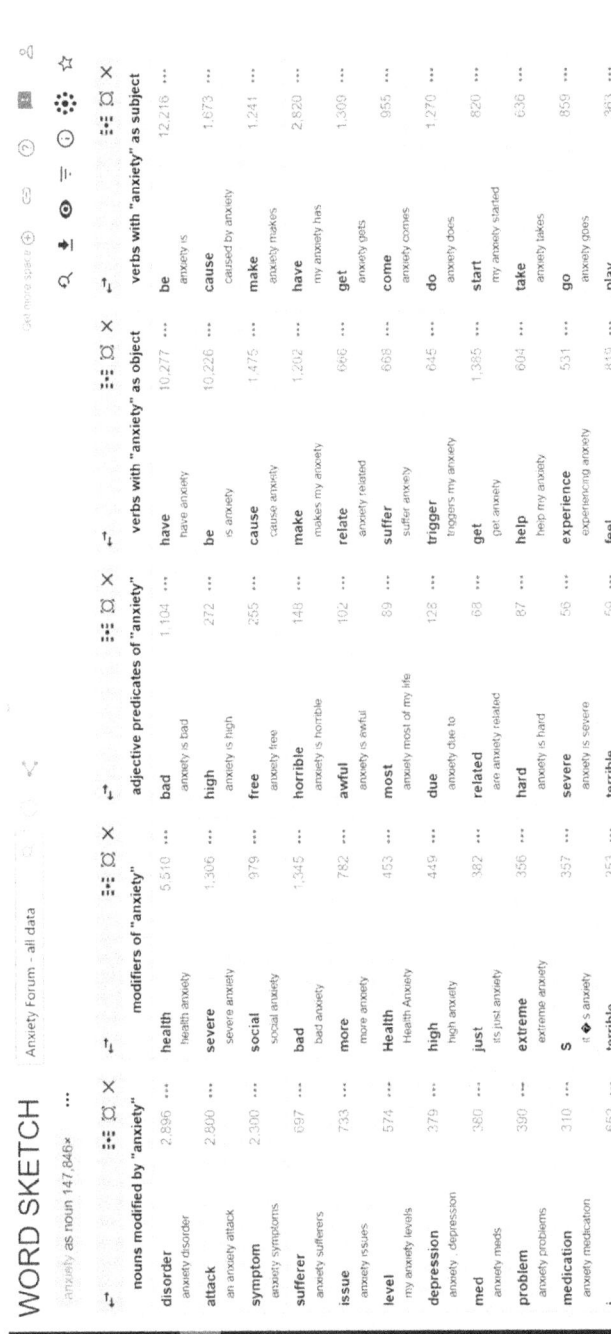

Figure 9.1 Word Sketch of *anxiety*.

also described as negative. But we should still bear in mind that these are separate (if related) representations, and not everything that is bad is a medical condition; some medical conditions can be seen as positive (e.g., genetic resistance to certain diseases, neurodiversity, or high pain tolerance).

9.2.2   Identifying Representations around Anxiety

The task of the researcher, then, is to consider the collocates in the Word Sketch and try to group them into ways that contribute towards discrete representations. Some words will be easier to categorise than others; some words might potentially contribute to more than one representation, depending on the context that they are used in; and for some words it might not be possible to identify a clear representation. The process of identifying categories and the words that go in them is therefore subjective, and it is unlikely that there will be a perfect way of doing it. It is important to try to apply a set of consistent and transparent guidelines when carrying out this kind of categorisation, and it is a good idea to work collaboratively, to help resolve difficult or ambiguous cases. While it is possible to categorise some words almost immediately (e.g., *bad*, *horrible*, and *awful* are fairly unambiguously negative), for other words, a detailed concordance analysis would be required. To be thorough, it is sensible to carry out concordance scans of all the words in the Word Sketch, just to confirm that a word is functioning in its expected way and something strange is not happening with it. Bear in mind, for example, that the Word Sketch shows all words in lowercase, but they might actually be realised with upper-case letters in the corpus. For instance, a word like *bad* could actually be an acronym (e.g., *BAD* can stand for a therapeutic approach known as behavioural activation for depression). In addition, negators may switch a collocate's meaning to its opposite – so in some cases people may write 'I don't have bad anxiety'.

As a result of grouping collocates together, the researchers identified four pairs of representations around anxiety, each pair of representations being related to one another. These pairs were (1) medicalising versus non-medicalising, (2) catastrophising versus minimising, (3) anthropomorphising versus abstracting, and (4) owning versus distancing. We will take the third pair as an example, in order to illustrate how these representations were realised through language.

Table 9.1 shows a range of ways that anxiety is metaphorically represented through language as a living being, often a human being but sometimes as an animal or a supernatural entity. This kind of representation casts anxiety as having agency, carrying out actions and having its own thoughts and goals.

In some cases anxiety was personified, through the use of prenominal titles like *Mr*, which occurs 34 times as a collocate of anxiety.

9.2 Representing Anxiety 139

Table 9.1 *Anthropomorphising representation of anxiety*

Structure	Examples
anxiety NOUN	bully (87), monster (36), demon (27), beast (13)
anxiety is a NOUN	beast (31), devil (30), bitch (22), culprit (17), enemy (17), liar (16), bully (15), monster (13), trickster (9), demon (9), tiger (8), fraud (9)
anxiety is not a NOUN	friend (10)
TITLE anxiety	Mr (34), Miss (1), Mrs (1)
anxiety VERB	cause (1,710), make (1,246), affect (273), try (249), hit (213), give (179), stop (114), create (109), bring (97), control (94), work (85), want (83), run (67), build (61), put (53), drive (45), like (48), let (45), produce (42), rule (43), provoke (40), need (46), love (40), lead (39), change (35), effect (29), mean (25), decide (23), send (21), prevent (21), rear (58), follow (36), take (641), suck (196), ruin (102), attack (91), feed (79), throw (47), hold (33), cripple (28), wake (26), rob (24), push (22), destroy (21), play (363), tell (167), think (120), act (72), talk (71), know (64), trick (46), mess (39), say (54), scare (29), bother (25), wait (24), exaggerate (23), convince (21), win (61), wear (29), beat (28), overwhelm (25), thrive (22)
VERB + anxiety	fight (316), beat (166), battle (80), conquer (60), tackle (51), combat (48), attack (32), challenge (24)

> **Mr Anxiety** has no regard for nice people or anyone eh?

A more common way that anxiety is anthropomorphised is by referring to it as a fantasy entity (*beast, devil, monster, demon*) or a malign human (*bitch, culprit, enemy, liar, bully, trickster, fraud*).

> **Anxiety** is a **beast** with a nature all it's own, but together we can learn to understand and embrace it for what it is

Table 9.1 also shows range of verb actions caried out by anxiety (verbs in their base form refer to all forms (e.g., *try* refers to *try, tries, tried*, and *trying*).

> when your **anxiety tries** to come knocking, remind it of today

> It's just **anxiety trying** to creep in.

Anxiety is also described as having conscious thoughts and desires, deciding, wanting, and loving things. Although *love* appears to be a positive word, it is used to describe anxiety as desiring negative outcomes for the person experiencing it.

> My **anxiety loves** to scare us and if you let it, its winning.

> right now my **anxiety wants** to rear its ugly head but I refuse to let it get me down

Anxiety is similarly described as playing tricks, scaring, and exaggerating.

> **Anxiety plays** mean tricks on the body so remember that

In addition, anxiety is assigned as the experiencer of the negative thought processes, as opposed to the person who experiences anxiety.

> That is your anxiety **thinking** negative thoughts.

A less common set of verbs involve descriptions of anxiety as beating the poster. These verbs often occur with negativisers (such as *no*, *not*, or *never*), where posters exhort one another or themselves not to let anxiety beat them.

> **Anxiety** well never **win** unless you let it.
>
> sometimes it's hard, but I'm not going to let this monster called **anxiety beat** me.

Other verbs in this representation describe anxiety as moving (*creep*, *follow*).

> I would say it's your health **anxiety following** you to the gym.
>
> Been fine all day come tea time felt **anxiety creeping** up on me.

Finally, there is a set of verbs which position anxiety as the patient of an action. Posters talk about *challenging*, *combatting*, *battling*, and *beating* anxiety. These kinds of verbs cast resolution of anxiety in terms of beating an opponent. In the following excerpt, the poster acknowledges the metaphorical nature of the representation by putting the word *weapons* in quote marks.

> As you know, there is no secret recipe for dealing with loss and tragedy, but providing yourself with an assortment of "weapons" to **combat the anxiety** is your best bet to defeat it!!

Viewing anxiety as a living being can be seen as management strategy for some posters. Chen, Chen, and Yang (2019) have described a study where individuals who were instructed to anthropomorphise sadness or happiness reported less experience of that emotion afterwards. They argue that the reduction of emotion occurs because anthropomorphic thinking increases the perceived distance between the self and the emotion, which results in a sense of detachment.

At other times, posters cast anxiety as an abstract state or entity (e.g., something which has no concrete state), as shown by the collocates in Table 9.2.

Rather than being a living or human entity, the words in this table represent anxiety through a range of different perspectives. For example, some posters metaphorically represent anxiety as an experience, journey, or story, which frames it as part of a person's life narrative.

> I guess we just have to accept it as a part of our **anxiety journey**

A less frequent category of words describe anxiety in terms of a negative and repetitive experience, using terms like *cycle*, *loop*, and *spiral*, a set of

9.2 Representing Anxiety

Table 9.2 *Anxiety as an abstract entity*

Structure	Examples
anxiety NOUN	disorder (2,913), issue (757), problem (398), thing (195), state (153), condition (56), stuff (40), side (33), part (33), journey (27), diagnosis (28), illness (23), experience (22), situation (21), bout (15), story (15), crap (14), struggle (14), relapse (13), shit (11), cycle (131), loop (38), spiral (25), trap (10)
anxiety is (a) NOUN	illness (76), problem (46), condition (32), issue (32), paradox (25), disorder (25), disease (18), habit (14), pain (28), hell (22), nightmare (19), game (15), circle (12), battle (10), trigger (11), bluff (10), trick (8), cycle (8), feeling (71), fear (71), thought (21), stress (13), reaction (12), emotion (12), response (10), thing (225), something (81), part (64), way (35), step (19), state (15), form (10)
anxiety VERB	kick (246), flare (66), increase (55), worsen (50), strike (33), kill (33), rise (29), grow (28), drain (28), heighten (27), reduce (24), decrease (22)
VERB anxiety	experience (536), feel (817), spike (23), lessen (72), alleviate (32), decrease (24)

characterisations which are linked to acknowledging that negative representations can result in increased anxiety.

> How do you stay positive and hopeful through this **anxiety spiral**?

> *Anxiety trap* works in a similar way.

> try focusing your attention on other things that can help you overcome the **anxiety trap**

In this category, words which involve increasing anxiety are also included, like *heighten, worsen, raise, escalate, add, exacerbate,* and *spike.* Again, these verbs are often used in explanatory contexts.

> The more we focus on our bodily functions it can **heighten** your **anxiety** and make you feel worse.

It can be useful to obtain a more general sense of a word's overall meaning by consulting a larger reference corpus. For example, *escalate* is used in the English Web 2020 Corpus to refer to abstract phenomena like *tension, violence, conflict, war, crisis, confrontation,* and *dispute* – it clearly has a semantic prosody for negative things, as well as abstract concepts.

> The **anxiety** just **escalates** it by a million percent.

Subside also has a semantic prosody for abstract entities. In the English Web 2020 Corpus, things that subside include *laughter, pain, swelling, anger, fever, storm, flood,* and *fighting.*

> I know when my **anxiety subsides** the symptoms will too.

Additionally, anxiety is represented as abstract negative phenomena – for example, as a repetitive process (*circle, cycle*), a place (*hell*), a bad dream (*nightmare*), or a contest (*battle, game*).

> **Anxiety** is **hell** on earth
>
> **Anxiety** is a **circle** and that is something we need to try to break out from.
>
> **Anxiety** is just as mind **game**, and games were meant to be won.

Coming somewhere between the abstracting and anthropomorphising representations of anxiety is a much smaller third set which frames anxiety as a non-living object. For example, there are verb metaphors like *fix* and *fuel* which cast anxiety as something akin to a machine.

> The fact that the medical profession only masks symptoms and has no conclusive understanding of the brain, basically means that you are paying for someone who has about as much chance as **fixing anxiety** as a plumber!!
>
> I keep googling symptoms too which is **fuelling my anxiety**.

Finally, there are another set of verbs, often denoting physical violence, which characterise anxiety even more negatively, as an entity which physically abuses the sufferer. It is difficult to categorise these verbs as referring to an abstract, living, or non-living entity, as they tend to occur in general language use in a wide range of contexts. Some of these verbs are used in metaphorical ways to describe anxiety as appearing or worsening (e.g., *kick in, flare, strike*). These verbs can also index natural phenomena. For example, in the English Web 2020 Corpus, *strike* tends to be associated with *lightning* or *earthquakes*, although there are also references to human-made objects (*bullet, missile, car*) or abstract concepts (*tragedy, disaster*) striking.

> sometimes **anxiety strikes** out of the blue for no reason
>
> it's not long before **anxiety** soon **kicks** in and wrecks everything again!

It is important to note that a single lexical item can invoke more than one kind of representation. For example, referring to anxiety as a disorder is a way of representing it as both an abstract concept and a medical condition, while calling anxiety a nightmare will represent it as an abstract concept and an extremely negative phenomena (a form of catastrophisation).

Identifying these kinds of representations is one stage of the analysis. We might want to consider the kinds of contexts that the different representations occur in. For example, the representations which describe anxiety as a living entity often tend to be used when posters provide one another with emotional support or advice on coping, while cases of catastrophisation of anxiety in the corpus tend to occur when people are seeking help. We may also want to consider which kinds of posters use certain types of representations (in terms of, say, demographic characteristics or the length of time they have spent on the forum). And we could also consider the ways that other posters respond to these representations: do they take them up themselves, reject them, or explicitly talk about their effectiveness in helping them resolve or manage their anxiety?

For medical practitioners, it could be argued that it is useful to have awareness of the ways that people use language to refer to anxiety. This could help practitioners reflect on the ways their clients represent anxiety and whether such representations are likely to help or hinder them. For example, there is some evidence that catastrophising is a positive predictor of anxiety (Chan et al., 2015). Practitioners could thus support clients in critically considering a range of possible representations of anxiety, helping them to shift their thinking about anxiety towards more constructive means. It should be borne in mind, however, that people are likely to respond differently to the same representation, so there will be no single ideal way of talking about anxiety that works for everyone. Instead, the analysis from the corpus of forum posts provides information about a range of possible representations and encourages awareness relating to the way that those representations impact our experience of health conditions. This sense of gaining a better understanding of the possible set of representations around illness, and their effects, continues in the following section.

9.3   Representing Cancer

In the previous section we showed how the corpus-based analysis of personal accounts of anxiety led to the identification of patterns of metaphor use that are relevant to understanding people's lived experience. We now turn to a corpus-based study that focused on metaphor specifically, in relation to cancer: the 'Metaphor in End-of-Life Care' project (MELC; Semino et al., 2018), already discussed in Chapter 5. Here we show how the analysis of a corpus of online forum posts by patients revealed the ways in which metaphors to do with violent encounters (e.g., fights and wars) are used to represent different aspects of the experience of having cancer.

The background and inspiration for this study was a long-standing debate on the dominance of what have been variously called 'war', 'military', 'fight', or 'battle' metaphors for cancer. Except for quotations, we will follow Semino and colleagues (2018) in subsuming all such metaphors under the label 'Violence' metaphors.

At the end of the 1970s, sociologist Susan Sontag (1979) famously objected to the use of what she called 'military' metaphors for being ill with cancer and tuberculosis, and argued for the elimination of metaphors from communication about cancer. Since then, Violence metaphors have been similarly criticised by patients, health professionals, and researchers from different disciplines (e.g., Miller, 2010; Granger, 2014). Critics pointed out that within these metaphors, the patient is either implicitly placed in the passive position of battleground or described as a fighter who is in an antagonistic relationship with the illness and thus their own body. Most importantly, within these metaphors, not recovering and eventually dying of cancer constitute 'losing the battle', which may suggest that the person is somehow responsible for their own condition and death. For example, Jane Granger, a UK doctor who was diagnosed with incurable cancer in her early 30s, wrote the following 2 years before her death:

> 'She lost her brave fight.' If anyone mutters those words after my death, wherever I am, I will curse them. ... I do not want to feel a failure about something beyond my control. I refuse to believe my death will be because I didn't battle hard enough. (Granger, 2014)

Indeed, policy documents in the UK, such as the 2007 *National Health Service Cancer Reform Strategy* (2007) and the *Cancer Strategy for England* (2015–20), have avoided military metaphors in policy documents and adopted instead the metaphor of the 'cancer journey', with different care 'pathways' for different patients.

It has also been pointed out that Violence metaphors can be highly meaningful and motivating for some patients. For example, Reisfield and Wilson (2004) discuss the case of a patient who, as a professional war historian, found military imagery particularly appropriate and used it extensively and creatively in his own correspondence. In a 2013 TED Talk, Amanda Bennett, a Pulitzer Prize–winning journalist whose husband died of cancer, argues for what she calls a 'heroic narrative of death', in which people with cancer and their families persist in hoping for a positive outcome until death (www.ted.com/talks/amanda_bennett_we_need_a_heroic_narrative_for_death?language=en).

In this context, the MELC team set out to use corpus methods to systematically analyse the ways in which metaphors generally, and Violence metaphors in particular, are used for the experience of cancer. The team then considered the implications of the findings for the experiences of patients in particular.

9.3.1 Creating a Cancer-Related Corpus and Identifying Metaphors

The MELC team collected a 1.5-million-word corpus consisting of interviews with and online writing by members of three stakeholder groups in cancer care: patients with cancer, unpaid family carers, and healthcare professionals. An overview of the MELC corpus is provided in Table 9.3 (Semino et al., 2018: 50). More specifically, the interviews involved

- 29 patients who had been diagnosed with advanced cancer (Payne et al., 2008);
- 17 unpaid carers who looked after a family member with a diagnosis of advanced cancer (Payne et al., 2009); and

9.3 Representing Cancer

Table 9.3 *Word counts in the MELC corpus*

	Patients	Unpaid family carers	Healthcare professionals	Totals
Semi-structured interviews	100,859	81,564	89,943	272,366
Contributions to online forums	500,134	500,256	253,168	1,253,558
Totals	**600,993**	**581,820**	**343,111**	**1,525,924**

- 16 senior healthcare professionals working in hospice or palliative care.

The online writing was produced in the period from 2007 to 2012 by

- 56 patients and 56 family carers writing on one particular UK-based online forum dedicated to cancer; and
- 307 healthcare professionals, writing on online forums or blogs.

The MELC corpus was too large to be analysed manually for the use of metaphor. On the other hand, no automated system for metaphor identification was deemed appropriate for the purposes of the project (e.g., Dunn, 2013). The team thus adopted a combination of manual and computational analysis. They created a sample corpus consisting of approximately 90,000 words (i.e., approximately 15,000 words from each of the six sections of the corpus outlined in Table 9.3) and employed existing metaphor identification procedures (Pragglejaz Group, 2007; Steen et al., 2010) to manually code this corpus for all instances of linguistic metaphors relevant to the experience of cancer. The linguistic metaphors were also tagged for the semantic domains that corresponded to their literal meanings – for example, Violence for 'battle', Journey for 'path' and Sports for 'marathon'. A tailor-made database was then employed to match the expressions included under each semantic grouping to the semantic domains in the USAS semantic tagger, which is implemented in the online corpus analysis tool Wmatrix (Rayson, 2008), as explained in Chapter 7.

More specifically, during the manual analysis of the sample corpus, the team classified as Violence metaphors

> any metaphorical expressions or similes whose literal meanings suggest scenarios in which, prototypically, a human agent intentionally causes physical harm to another human, with or without weapons. Less prototypical scenarios involve non-human agents, the threat or consequences of violence, or non-physical harm. (Semino et al., 2018: 100)

The linguistic metaphors that fit this definition were then matched with the corresponding USAS semantic tags in Wmatrix by means of the database mentioned earlier. This revealed that the following USAS semantic domains included expressions that could be used metaphorically to describe the experience of cancer in terms of various kinds of violent encounters (Semino et al., 2018: 100):

- G3 (Warfare): for example, *fight* as a verb; *battle*
- E3– (Violent/angry): for example, *hit*; *attack*
- S8+ (Helping): for example, *defend*; *protect*
- S8– (Hindering): for example, *fight* as a noun
- X8+ (Trying hard): for example, *struggle*
- A1.1.1 (General actions, making): for example, *blast* and *confront*
- A1.1.2 (Damaging and destroying): for example, *destroy*; *shatter*

The team then analysed all concordance lines for each of these semantic domains in the complete corpus and identified all instances where the relevant lexical item was used metaphorically to capture some aspect of the experience of cancer. The use of semantic domain concordances meant that it was possible to identify metaphorical expressions that did not occur in the sample corpus. This does not of course mean that *all* Violence metaphors in the analysis would have been captured. However, as described in the following sections, a substantial number of instances were identified, and the fact that the same approach was adopted for all sections of the corpus also means that comparisons were possible.

9.3.2 Violence Metaphors and Different Stakeholder Groups

In this section we report the most relevant findings with regard to Violence metaphors. We begin with quantitative findings and then move on to qualitative observations.

The MELC team found that Violence and Journey metaphors were the most frequently used types of metaphors in all sections of the corpus (Semino et al., 2018: 84) and that Violence metaphors were the most frequently used by patients in particular.

Table 9.4 and Figure 9.2 (from Semino et al., 2018: 101–2) provide raw and normalised frequencies for Violence metaphors in the three groups of people and two genres included in the MELC corpus.

Violence metaphors are used by members of all three groups in both genres. However, in the online data, patients use Violence metaphors more frequently than family carers and healthcare professionals, with 1.8 instances per 1,000 words versus 1.61 and 1.33, respectively, for carers and professionals. Semino and colleagues (2018: 102) report that this difference across the three groups is statistically significant (using a log likelihood test for uniformity: $p < 0.05$, 2 d.f., log likelihood = 23.22).

9.3 Representing Cancer

Table 9.4 *Distribution of Violence metaphors in the MELC corpus*

	Patients		Unpaid family carers		Healthcare professionals		All groups combined	
	RF	NF	RF	NF	RF	NF	RF	NF
Interviews	72	0.71	80	0.98	73	0.81	225	0.83
Online forum posts	899	1.80	807	1.61	337	1.33	2043	1.63
Interviews and online forum posts combined	971	1.62	887	1.52	410	1.19	2268	1.49

RF, raw frequency; NF, normalised frequencies per 1,000 words.

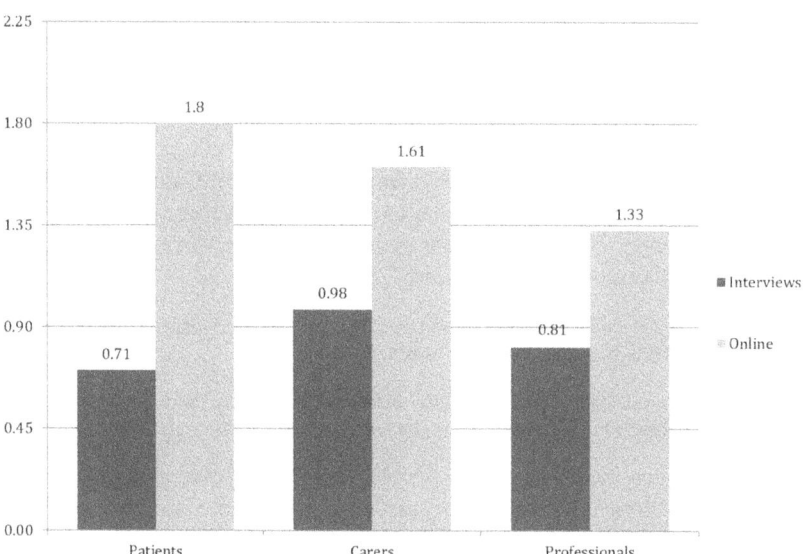

Figure 9.2 Frequencies of Violence metaphors in the corpus per 1,000 words.

The MELC team considered all instances of Violence metaphors in order to establish *how* they are used in context. This led to two main findings. First, there is no single Violence or War metaphor where the disease is an enemy that needs to fought by the patient or by healthcare professionals, as implicitly suggested by previous literature. On the contrary, patients in particular use Violence metaphors to talk about different aspects of their experience of illness, including the relationship with cancer, the effects of treatment, and the patients' relationship with the healthcare system. Second, while there is evidence in the

MELC corpus of the potentially harmful consequences of Violence metaphors, there is also evidence that they can be meaningful and motivating for some patients, at least some of the time. The MELC team expressed this contrast in terms of the concept of '(dis)empowerment', defined as 'the process through which linguistic choices reflect, facilitate and/or undermine different kinds and degrees of agency, validation, evaluation and control, with implications for identities, emotions and relationships' (Semino et al., 2018: 7).

Whether a Violence metaphor or, in fact, any metaphor is empowering or disempowering depends on who uses it and how in a specific context (Semino et al., 2017).

In the next section we consider the different aspects of the cancer experience that patients use Violence metaphors for in the MELC data, with special emphasis on the contrast between empowering and disempowering uses (Semino et al., 2018: 105ff.).

9.3.3 Violence Metaphors and Different Aspects of Patients' Experiences with Cancer

Violence metaphors are used by some patients in the MELC corpus to portray their relationship with cancer as antagonistic and competitive, and to express their determination to recover. These are the kinds of Violence metaphors that had been the focus of previous studies:

> I don't intend to give up; I don't intend to give in. No I want to fight it. I don't want it to beat me, I want to beat it.

> I have not hunkered down in my trench to just merely defend myself against the demon but have picked up my sword and taken the fight to the demon

In both examples, the patient places themselves in an empowered position; they present themselves as active and focussed, and as hopeful about their outlook.

The potential for Violence metaphors to be used in empowering ways is particularly evident when patients describe themselves as *fighters*:

> I was also fortunate that my Consultants recognised that I was a born fighter and saw my determination

This metaphorical use of *fighter* does not so much evoke an oppositional scenario with the illness as the enemy but rather presents the person as optimistic and ready to do everything they can to get better (cf. *determination* in the provided extract).

Semino and colleagues (2018) also notice that some empowering uses of Violence metaphors involve humour, as mentioned in Chapter 5:

> Don't let the Demon get you down, spit it in it's eye and give it a swift kick up the wahoola.

9.3 Representing Cancer

Here the cancer is menacingly described as a 'Demon', but the use of 'wahoola' as part of a Violence metaphor involving physical struggle makes light of what is otherwise a serious situation. The cancer is personified as the butt of the joke, thereby placing the patient in the empowered position of making fun of the illness. The MELC team showed more broadly how this kind of humour was employed by patients in the online data to release tension, demystify the illness, and strengthen the social bonds among contributors to the forum (Semino et al., 2018: 233ff.; see also Semino and Demjén, 2017).

In contrast, when Violence metaphors are used to express the fear or prospect of not recovering, the patient is placed in a disempowered position:

> I feel such a failure that I am not winning this battle

> I sometimes worry about being so positive or feel I am being cocky when I say I will fight this as I think oh my god what if I don't win people will think ah see I knew she couldn't do it!

In both examples provided, not getting better (and therefore potentially dying of cancer), is metaphorically described as 'not winning', as part of Violence metaphors (cf. *battle* and *fight* in the extracts provided). In addition, in both cases, the person suggests that they feel responsible for not recovering or anticipates that others will see them as responsible. This is where Violence metaphors can do harm, as suggested by their critics. In a violent confrontation – whether a physical struggle or a battle between armies – the party that is defeated is typically perceived to weaker, less determined, or less well organised. Within a violence framing for illness, these associations are attributed to the person who does not recover, resulting in the person feeling 'a failure' or anticipating embarrassment for not getting better, when in fact they bear no responsibility for the course of their illness.

In the following example, in contrast, the patient is implicitly disempowered in relation to the healthcare system, as they are not being provided with the treatment (*armour*) that they believe they need to get better:

> it must be dispiriting when you are battling as hard as you can, not to be given the armour to fight in

The MELC team noticed that the term *battle*, as a noun or as a verb, had a tendency to be used to suggest disempowerment, either because of extreme difficulties experienced by patients or the unsuccessful outcome of treatment (Semino et al., 2018: 109).

While it was previously known that Violence metaphors were frequently used to talk about having cancer and trying to get better, the analysis of the MELC corpus also revealed the use of Violence metaphors for the effects that cancer treatment has on the patient. In such cases the violence-related metaphorical expressions evoke scenarios dealing with personal physical aggression, such as 'a battering from chemo', 'a "hammering" from medication', or various uses of the verb 'hit':

> They hit me with radiation for 10 days.
>
> what did i think all my normal little cells were doing after being hit by a sledgehammer of both toxic chemicals and radiation

Here the process of being treated with radiotherapy and/or chemotherapy is presented as being on the receiving end of a violent attack. The emphasis is not so much on 'losing' against the aggressor but on the damage that results from the attack, especially where the metaphorical expressions suggest extreme violence, as in the case of 'hit by a sledgehammer'. Cancer treatment is well known to have major side effects, especially in the case of chemotherapy. The use of Violence metaphors for treatment suggests the seriousness of these side effects while also conveying a sense of helplessness and disempowerment in the context of medical interventions that are intended to help the person recover or live longer.

The analysis of the MELC corpus also revealed instances of Violence metaphors where the two opponents were the patient and the healthcare system:

> that first lady that was well publicised about fighting and getting the Herceptin
>
> I will fight for Avastin.

These uses of Violence metaphors reflect the perception of difficulty and effort involved in obtaining the treatment that the patients feel they need. With regard to (dis)empowerment, on the one hand the patients place themselves in the active position of agents advocating for themselves. However, they are not in fact empowered, partly for having to argue for their own treatment at a point of extreme vulnerability, and partly because the decision-making power with regard to that treatment ultimately lies with health professionals and policy makers.

As we showed in Chapter 5, a different use of Violence metaphors for the patient's relationship with the health system involves empowerment through humour (Semino et al., 2018: 252–5). A group of contributors to a particular thread dedicated to cancer-related humour describe themselves as a small army aiming to 'liberate' specific individuals from the hospital and even give each other military titles and promotions to higher ranks. This long-running collaborative joke shows the power of the combination of metaphor and humour to create distance, at least temporarily, from a situation of hardship, and to foster emotional closeness with others in the same situation.

Overall, the use of corpus methods to systematically study the Violence metaphors used by patients revealed a greater variety of uses than had been previously noticed. Among other things, this shows how patients may feel in a situation where they are 'fighting' on several fronts – against the illness, against the treatment, and against the healthcare system. On the other hand, while Violence metaphors can be disempowering, they can also be used in empowering ways, especially when they are combined with humour.

9.4 Conclusion

It matters if you talk about anxiety in terms of having an illness or disease or if you say you are an anxious kind of person. And it matters if you view cancer in terms of battling it or as going on a journey. This chapter has offered two techniques for analysing the ways that patients understand health conditions and their relationship to them, arguably an important component of helping patients understand, accept, and manage those conditions. The first was focused on identifying different representations around a single word in a corpus (anxiety); the second involved analysing an entire corpus while focusing on a difficult-to-find linguistic phenomenon (metaphor). Both techniques utilised quantitative and qualitative approaches, using corpus tools like Word Sketch (Sketch Engine) and Wmatrix, which were then combined with more detailed analyses of concordance lines and consideration of context. In the following chapter, we continue the consideration of representation but now move away from health conditions to the people who experience them.

References

Chan, S. M., Chan, S. K. and Kwok, W. W. (2015). Ruminative and Catastrophizing Cognitive Styles Mediate the Association between Daily Hassles and High Anxiety in Hong Kong Adolescents. *Child Psychiatry and Human Development*, 46, 57–66. https://doi.org/10.1007/s10578-014-0451-9.

Chen, F., Chen, R. P. and Yang, L. (2019). When Sadness Comes Alive, Will It Be Less Painful? The Effects of Anthropomorphic Thinking on Sadness Regulation and Consumption. *Journal of Consumer Psychology*, 30(2), 277–95. https://doi.org/10.1002/jcpy.1137.

Collins, L. and Baker, P. (2023). *Language, Discourse and Anxiety*. Cambridge University Press.

Dunn, J. (2013). Evaluating the Premises and Results of Four Metaphor Identification Systems. In A. Gelbukh (ed.), *Proceedings of CICLing 2013, LNCS 7816* (pp. 471–86). Springer.

Granger, K. (2014). Having Cancer Is Not a Fight or a Battle. *The Guardian*. www.theguardian.com/society/2014/apr/25/having-cancer-not-fight-or-battle. Accessed 14 December 2024.

Miller, R. S. (2010). Speak Up: 8 Words and Phrases to Ban in Oncology! *Oncology Times*, 32(12), 20. https://doi.org/10.1097/01.COT.0000383777.50536.b2.

Payne, S., Chapman, A., Froggatt, K., Gott, M. and Chung, M. (2008). *Ethnicity and Cancer: Examining Psychosocial Transitions for Older People*. Final report. Dimbleby Cancer Care.

Payne, S., Ingleton, C., Nolan, M. and O'Brien, T. (2009). *Evaluation of the Help the Hospices Major Grants Programme for Carers of Those Who Are Terminally Ill*. Final report. Help the Hospices.

Pragglejaz Group (2007). MIP: A Method for Identifying Metaphorically Used Words in Discourse. *Metaphor and Symbol*, *22*(1), 1–39. https://doi.org/10.1080/10926480709336752.

Rayson, P. (2008). From Key Words to Key Semantic Domains. *International Journal of Corpus Linguistics*, *13*(4), 519–49. https://doi.org/10.1075/ijcl.13.4.06ray.

Reisfield, G. M. and Wilson, G. R. (2004). Use of Metaphor in the Discourse on Cancer. *Journal of Clinical Oncology*, *22*(19), 4024–7. https://doi.org/10.1200/JCO.2004.03.136.

Semino, E. and Demjén, Z. (2017). The Cancer Card: Metaphor, Intimacy and Humour in Online Interactions about the Experience of Cancer. In B. Hampe (ed.), *Metaphor: Embodied Cognition & Discourse* (pp. 181–99). Cambridge University Press.

Semino, E., Demjén, Z., Demmen, J., Koller, V., Payne, S., Hardie, H. and Rayson, P. (2017). The Online Use of 'Violence' and 'Journey' Metaphors by Cancer Patients, as Compared with Health Professionals: A Mixed Methods Study. *BMJ Supportive and Palliative Care*, *7*(1), 60–6. https://doi.org/10.1136/bmjspcare-2014-000785.

Semino, E., Demjén, Z., Hardie, A., Rayson, P. and Payne, S. (2018). *Metaphor, Cancer and the End of Life: A Corpus-based Study*. Routledge.

Sontag, S. (1979). *Illness as Metaphor*. Allen Lane.

Steen, G. J., Dorst, A. G., Herrmann, B. J., Kaal, A. A., Krennmayr, T. and Pasma, T. (2010). *A Method for Linguistic Metaphor Identification: From MIP to MIPVU*. John Benjamins.

Stubbs, M. (2001). *Words and Phrases*. Blackwell.

10 Representing Social Actors

10.1 Introduction

We can think of healthcare as a constellation of social practices: as the repeated performance of actions determined by the co-constitutive relationship between structure and individual agency (Giddens, 1984). In other words, individuals can make decisions that impact their health, such as going to see the doctor for advice and treatment and manging their diet and exercise, but healthcare outcomes equally depend on structural effects, such as the availability of treatments, nutritious food, or facilities that enable active lifestyles. Structural aspects and individual (health) choices are co-constitutive in that one determines the other (Maller, 2015). By conceptualising healthcare in terms of social practices, we can posit the various stakeholders (i.e., health practitioners, patients, governments, business owners, news writers etc.) as social actors – agents that play a key role in creating our social world, including how healthcare is delivered.

Studies of social actor representation have typically drawn on Van Leeuwen's (1996) influential social actor network, in which he describes the various strategies through which participants are foregrounded or backgrounded when they are identified in the text or otherwise excluded entirely. For example, social actors can be described according to their functional role or physical characteristics, and individuals can be marked out independently or presented as part of a collective. In short, the key question driving social actor analysis can be expressed as Darics and Koller (2019: 224) posit in their framework: 'How are social actors represented: as active or passive, as more or less agentive, and in personal or impersonal ways?'

Relatedly, we can consider what participants are represented as *doing* as indicative of their role and their capacity to contribute to the delivery of healthcare. One of the concepts through which researchers have investigated the actions and behaviours that social actors are involved in is 'transitivity', and transitivity analysis offers a framework for classifying processes that assists us in pointing to different levels of agency (Halliday and Matthiessen, 2014). Furthermore, if we posit that representations of social actors are choices, consistent with the principles of the wider conceptual framework for systemic functional linguistics, we can consider the selection of particular naming strategies and reported actions in relation to the institutional and social contexts in which they appear. Or, as Van Leeuwen (2008: 33) asks, 'What interests are served by them, and what purposes achieved?'

In this chapter, we demonstrate how corpus approaches assisted us in examining the representation of social actors: first, in UK media coverage of people with obesity and, second, in interview responses provided by participants with psychosis, leading them to hear voices that others cannot. Through discussion of these case studies, we will show how recurrent naming strategies contribute to the stigmatisation of people with obesity and how the actions ascribed to voices demonstrates how voice-hearers navigate experiences that are often distressing. Ultimately, we will show that there are steps in the analysis of social actors that can be supported by the computationally driven procedures of corpus analysis, while other aspects are better suited to the more contextualised and discerning reading provided by the informed analyst.

10.2 Representing Obesity in the British National Press

In this section we describe how members of the CASS team identified representations of people with obesity in a 36-million-word corpus of British newspaper articles about obesity published between 2008 and 2017 (see Brookes and Baker, 2021, and Sections 2.3, 3.2, and 7.2 of this book). The articles were collected using the LexisNexis online news database, with the stipulation that they had to contain at least one mention of the word *obese* or *obesity*. The researchers had conducted similar types of research on newspaper discourse in the past. For example, Baker and co-authors (2013) examined a 140-million-word corpus of news articles about Muslims and Islam. They examined representations by conducting collocation and concordance analyses around a small set of relevant words like *Muslim*, *Muslims*, *Islam*, and *Islamic*. However, when examining the corpus of articles about obesity, it was not as easy to focus the analysis on a few words, as initial examination of samples of articles indicated that people with obesity were referred to in a wide number of ways, ranging from positive to neutral to euphemistic to explicitly stigmatising.

10.2.1 Social Actors in Obesity Coverage

In their analysis, Brookes and Baker (2021) incorporated Reisgl and Wodak's discourse historical approach (2001), which like social actor analysis considers referential/nomination and predication strategies. The former pertains to how individuals are named and referred to, while the latter deals with how they are described and what qualities or characteristics are attributed to them.

10.2 Representing Obesity in the British National Press

A nomination strategy might involve using a noun like *fatso*, while a predication strategy could include adjectives like *pathetic* or verbs describing certain actions (e.g., *wolfing down food*) or being the recipient of actions (e.g., *labelled as obese*).

Additionally, Brookes and Baker (2021) utilised Van Leeuwen's (1996) social actor representation framework, which offers a system for categorizing the ways that social actors are portrayed in English discourse. For instance, terms like *the obese* involve physical identification, uniquely defining individuals based on their physical characteristics within a given context. This framework helped researchers identify how references to people with obesity can either include or exclude, personalise or impersonalise, assimilate or differentiate them in the discourse. The researchers uploaded the corpus into the online analysis tool CQPweb (Hardie, 2012), so the analysis described in the following section uses the search facilities associated with that tool, although other tools should allow for similar kinds of searches to be carried out.

10.2.2 Nomination Strategies

The analysis began with the identification of nomination strategies. Once a set of those were found, Brookes and Baker (2021) could then more easily find the predication strategies through the consideration of collocates and concordance lines. Identifying nomination strategies was not a simple task, however, and the researchers employed several non-corpus-assisted and corpus-assisted tactics in order to produce a list.

The two main non-corpus-assisted methods involved using introspection and reading samples of articles from the corpus. The researchers asked friends, family members, and colleagues to think of possible terms that might appear in the corpus, in order to triangulate from different perspectives. Subsequent to the completion of the study, the researchers decided to see whether a tool like ChatGPT would have been useful for identifying further terms. ChatGPT initially offered a list of terms that it described as 'neutral and descriptive', like *person with a higher body mass*. Its initial response was lightly chastising, stating: 'Remember to use language that is respectful and non-stigmatizing when discussing individuals' weight or body size.' However, when the purpose of the study was explained in more detail, ChatGPT produced a wider list of words which included stigmatising ones like *whale* and *blob*.

The corpus-assisted methods of eliciting nominations involved the examination of frequency and keyword lists. The researchers identified keywords for each newspaper by using 'the remainder method' (i.e., comparing a frequency list of articles from a single newspaper against a reference corpus consisting of the remaining newspaper articles they had collected; see Chapter 7). This helped identify terms that tended to be popular in a single paper. For instance, nouns like *fatties* and *flab* were prominent in *The Star* compared to the other newspapers in the corpus. The researchers also tried to identify relatively infrequent nouns in each newspaper by looking at wordlists. For example, when they obtained a frequency list of *The Times*, they looked at plural nouns that occurred between 4 and 10 times in the corpus. This produced words like *bloaters*, *heavyweights*, and *overeaters*, which had not been identified by any other means.

10.2.3 Collocation Analysis

Once they had an initial set of words, Brookes and Baker (2021) identified collocates, focussing particularly on adjectival and verb collocates, as these were most likely to reveal predication strategies. These collocates also provided an additional route for finding new nominations. For example, when examining collocates of *slob*, the researchers found adjectives like *fat*, *boozy*, *lazy*, and *out-of-shape*. Conducting searches of these adjectives and examining words which collocated with them produced additional nomination labels like *lard-arse*, *hog*, *porker*, *lump*, and *fatty*. As they conducted their analyses, the researchers kept an open eye when reading concordance lines, in order to identify further terms. This meant that they had to regularly update frequency tables as new terms were elicited during the analysis.

The researchers were working with a grammatically tagged version of the corpus, which allowed them to easily expand the analysis to account for both singular and plural forms of nouns (e.g., *slob*, *slobs*), as well as comparative and superlative forms of adjectives (e.g., *chunky*, *chunkier*, *chunkiest*) and related verb tenses (e.g., *guzzle*, *guzzles*, *guzzled*, *guzzling*). Within CQPweb, putting a search word within curly brackets retrieves all its related grammatical forms. For instance, searching for {waddle/V} would elicit cases of *waddle*, *waddles*, *waddling*, and *waddled* as verbs.

For some terms, searches elicited a large number of false positives (i.e., unwanted cases). For example, the word *fat* often referred to the amount of fat in food. The researchers could search just for adjectival cases (tagged JJ), using the search query fat_JJ, although this still produced a high number of noun cases that were erroneously tagged as adjectives. Other cases used *fat* to modify nouns that did not refer to human beings (e.g., *fat crisis, fat gene, fat camp*). There were 22,578 cases of *fat* tagged as an adjective, so in order to obtain a reasonable estimation of the number of times the word *fat* appeared as an adjective which referred to a human being, the researchers carried out a qualitative examination of 10 per cent of concordance lines of fat_JJ, presented in random order (2,258 cases). They then multiplied the number of cases that referred to people by 10. Another set of unwanted cases involved the phrase *the obese*, which sometimes occurred as a collective noun but also often occurred as part of a longer noun phrase, such as *the obese singer.* A similar strategy to *fat* was used to isolate only the cases where *the obese* was used as a collective. This term only occurred 1,703 times in the corpus, so it was possible to carry out a concordance scan of all cases and remove cases like *the obese singer*, which didn't apply.

The researchers also obtained the collocates of a set of nouns that more generally referred to human beings (e.g., *people, men, women, children, kids, boys*, and *girls*), as these words sometimes occurred as parts of noun phrases relating to obesity (e.g., *obese people, supersize kids*). Different collocational statistics are likely to produce different kinds of findings. For example, the log ratio and mutual information statistics tended to produce low-frequency collocates which would point to rare nominations (e.g., *super-obese* is a top log-ratio collocate of *people*, occurring 11 times in the corpus). On the other hand, log likelihood foregrounded more frequent collocates like *obese*, which co-occurred with *people* 3,714 times.

In order to consider representation beyond simple noun labels, the researchers aimed to find a list of adjectives and verbs that tended to be used to refer to people with obesity in the corpus of news articles. Once they had identified a list of nominations, it was possible to obtain collocates for each one. As there were a large number of terms, comprising both singular and plural forms, a short cut to obtaining lists of adjective and verb collocates was to combine searches on multiple words in CQPweb. For example, researchers can put a number of similar terms within brackets, separating them with the | symbol, to consider them together:

(pig_NN1|hog_NN1|fatty_NN1|slob_NN1|porky_NN1|overweight people)

Researchers can then obtain the collocates of these collated terms, which would save time compared with having to conduct separate searches on each word. The researchers checked the resulting concordance lines of collocates to remove false positives. For example, based on the search query provided, the top-10 collocates (using log ratio) are *hydroxyl, Peppa, 'Oi, suckling, guinea, Percy, Daddy, salty,* and *metabolise*. Most of these collocates are modifying non-human cases such as *hydroxyl fatty acids* and *Peppa Pig*, and thus would need to be removed completely or at least have their frequencies adjusted.

10.2.4 Predication Strategies

Once Brookes and Baker (2021) had removed the false positives, they were able to obtain a list of adjectives used to refer to people with obesity, which was illuminating in revealing typical qualities that are associated with them. The researchers grouped the adjectives into categories which related to attractiveness (e.g., *ugly, beautiful*), health (*ill, unfit*), emotional state (*depressed, happy*), level of activity (*lazy*), intelligence (*stupid*), or other qualities (*funny, proud*). However, the researchers also wanted to identify adjectives that refer more directly to obesity as opposed to other qualities, such as *tubby, solid*, and *expansive*. Adjectives such as these can appear as predicative (e.g., *he is tubby*), and when attributive, they might not necessarily modify nouns relating to obesity but rather occur with general nouns like *person* or *man*. Again, a number of retrieval strategies were employed in order to obtain a list of these adjectives: introspection, reading samples, concordance lines, and through prospective collocation searches on relevant nouns or pronouns.

Once they had obtained a list of these adjectives, the researchers categorised them into those which were positive, euphemistic, or directly insulting towards people with obesity. One additional aspect of these adjectives that emerged as the researchers collected them was that some of them seemed to be gender-specific (e.g., *voluptuous* and *curvy* were used to refer to women with obesity, while *beefy* and *portly* referred to men with obesity), so the researchers noted such cases accordingly. Further, they noted that many of these words were often used alliteratively. For example, of the 125 references to *porky*, 63 (50.4 per cent) were followed by another word beginning with *p* (e.g., *pooch, pets, PCs, pupils*, etc.). Similar alliterative patterns are found with the other euphemistic adjectives (e.g., *chubby children, tubby toddlers, lardy lags, hefty hounds, flabby felines, voluptuous vixens*). Such cases are more typical of tabloid newspapers, which often use literary devices to make headlines more eye-catching. However, in terms of representing people, it could be argued that this alliterative language can result in a fictionalising effect, encouraging readers to think about the subjects as caricatures and distancing them from thinking about them as actual human beings.

Using collocates, the researchers also obtained lists of verbs that were used to modify references to people with obesity. Verbs were classified into groups which referred to

- food being consumed quickly and in large quantities (e.g., *gorge, scoff, cram, shovel*);
- ungainly movement (*lumber, waddle, jiggle*);
- discomfort (*sweat, wheeze*);
- weight gain (*balloon, pile on*); and
- difficulty fitting into space (*cram, wedge, clog, squeeze*).

These verbs were considered further in terms of the metaphors that they implied – for example, the verbs related to eating sometimes represented people with obesity as animal-like (e.g., *wolf, swill, pig out*). The researchers also considered verbs that positioned people with obesity as patients of actions, as opposed to agents. (The Sketch Engine analysis tool has a Word Sketch function that can make this distinction automatically; see Chapter 9.) This led the researchers to a small set of verb collocates like *brand, dub*, and *shame*, which were often used in sympathetic articles about people with obesity, where

10.2 Representing Obesity in the British National Press

they were sometimes presented as objects of pity or were the subject of redemptive weight-loss narratives. For example,

> Tubby teen to trolley dolly: Junk food addict **branded** "fat friend" on girls' holiday sheds 6st and lands job as air stewardess. (*Mirror*, 29 March 2017)

This mention of narratives points to a further, more qualitative stage of the analysis, which extends beyond identifying collocates to consider the wider contexts in which people with obesity are involved. This can be a less systematic form of analysis to engage in, and even a concordance line analysis may not be especially productive, requiring analysts to expand concordance lines to read entire texts to obtain a sense of the narrative structure of a particular article. Continuing with the redemptive weight-loss narratives, for example, the researchers found a pattern whereby numerous news articles (particularly in tabloids) told a real-life story about an individual (often an ordinary member of the public, although sometimes a celebrity) who had been bullied in childhood for being overweight and had gone on to lose a lot of weight as a result of a particular diet or exercise regime. The individual was described as having undergone an amazing and positive transformation, both physically and in terms of achieving success in other areas of their life. Such stories were somewhat formulaic, although the researchers also noted what they did *not* include, such as criticism of the bullies or acknowledgement that many people who lose a lot of weight quickly are likely to regain it after a few years. These narratives are therefore perhaps both inspiring and misleading to readers.

Alongside these narratives, the researchers' more detailed readings of concordance lines helped them identify two other ways that people with obesity were represented – as subject to ridicule and criminals. For example, they found a number of cases involving stories of convicted criminals who were described as having obesity:

> BEHIND BARS; Evil Huntley clinically obese after guzzling chocolates. SOHAM killer Ian Huntley has ballooned to almost 18 stone after bingeing on Wispa and Toffee Crisp chocolate bars in his cell. The 35-year-old monster is now clinically obese and is nicknamed "Blobby" by fellow lags. (*Star*, 31 May 2009)

This article observes Huntley's weight gain, portraying it as deserving public attention. However, reporting on his weight gain is tinged with a sense of delight, which, considering the overall media stance on weight gain, may be interpreted as a form of fitting retribution (with the article labelling Huntley as *evil* and *a monster*). The *Sun* article also implicitly links weight gain and crime, and the researchers also found articles that referred to people whose criminal behaviour was described as being directly related to their obesity:

> Obese woman who went on TV to complain that she was too fat to get a job caught stealing cakes just hours after This Morning appearance. (*Mail*, 29 March 2013)

Such stories collectively contribute to the portrayal of individuals with obesity as clumsy, petty wrongdoers, associating negative traits like greed and laziness with their weight. Consequently, these narratives contribute to depicting people with obesity in a comedic role. While the crimes of individuals like Huntley are not presented as humorous, stories about their weight gain are portrayed more frivolously, demonstrating the scope within which obesity is presented as subject for ridicule. Although such stories are not as prevalent as the weight-loss narratives mentioned earlier in this section, their frequency is sufficient to identify a pattern. The casual association of crime with obesity arguably represents one of the most unfavourable forms of representation in the corpus.

In summary, the case study described in this section indicates how representations can be found in corpora by beginning with the idea of nomination and nouns, and gradually expanding the remit to include predicative and attributive adjectives, as well as verbs which position social actors as agents or patients. We also saw how the analysis was expanded further to consider metaphors, gendered language, and stylistic features like alliteration, and then finally went beyond the lexis to explore narratives. In doing so, the analysis moved from the quantitative to the qualitative. While it cannot be said that every form of representation of people with obesity in the corpus has been identified, what the approach taken here does offer is a representative picture in order to draw meaningful and reasonable conclusions, while also allowing the researchers to provide information about the frequencies of different kinds of representations in comparison to one another.

10.3 Investigating the Agency of Voices in Psychosis

Our second case study concerns the experience of auditory verbal hallucinations (AVHs), commonly referred to as 'voices', as a kind of psychosis that is associated with mental health conditions such as schizophrenia, bipolar disorder, and borderline personality disorder (Woods et al., 2022). Such hallucinations are defined as 'sensory perceptions in the absence of any externally generated stimulus' (Lindenmayer and Khan, 2006: 198) or, to put it another way, an individual's perception of voices that others cannot hear. There are issues with the terms 'voices' and auditory verbal hallucinations, since these experiences can manifest in ways that are not 'heard' (Wilkinson and Bell, 2016). Nevertheless, in the absence of a suitable alternative, we adhere to the convention among researchers in the field, and indeed generally among those with lived experience, to use the term 'voices' to capture stimuli that might be otherwise described as ambient rather than communicative (e.g., *buzz*) or as some other sensation (e.g., *flashing, shaking*).

Voices in psychotic disorders are typically distressing and cause disruption in the lives of those who experience them, though interactions between the voice-hearer and their voices can range in their complexity and affect (Woods et al., 2022). Subsequently, there is growing interest in the ways that voices are personified and represented as social agents (see Wilkinson and Bell, 2016). It was on this basis that CASS researchers saw a way for language-based models of agency and social actor representation to contribute to mapping out the interpersonal mechanisms of voice-hearing. In what follows, we discuss transitivity as a system through which analysts can document the agency of social actors as it is demonstrated through processes. We reflect on aspects of existing frameworks that require some decision-making on the part of the analyst when applied to language data in context and consider how corpus procedures can assist in such investigations.

10.3.1 Hearing the Voice: Interviews with People Experiencing Psychosis

The data for this study were collected by the Hearing the Voice (HtV) team, operating in northeast England and carrying out work to better understand how voice-hearing experiences change over time (Woods et al., 2022). The HtV team interviewed volunteers who had sought support from local early intervention in psychosis services for their voices, and those interviews were transcribed and made available to CASS researchers for (corpus) linguistic analysis. Participants were given pseudonyms, and other personal information was anonymised. Forty individuals took part in semi-structured interviews with the HtV team, describing what their voices are like, when they started, what they do and say, and how they have changed over time. This amounted to 205,941 words of participant data that the CASS team compiled and analysed as a corpus.

One of the objectives of the HtV team was to investigate the personification of the reported voices and how this varies according to degrees of complexity. This aim was predicated on the understanding that voices can variously be attributed attitudes, intentions, and different kinds of identities (even names). They can also manifest as other non-human (*demon, birds, bomb*) or abstract entities (*thoughts, scenario, sensation*). The HtV team established a binary classification for manually coding the reported voices in terms of the complexity of personification, according to the following definitions:

Minimal personification: The voice has few person-like qualities; is attributed to a person or described as being 'like a person' but without further elaboration. Person-like characteristics tend to remain stable over time and follow a single theme (e.g., the voice is 'mean', or a 'nasty man').

Complex personification: The voice is described as having more than one kind of person-like quality. These may include elaborate descriptions of intentional states (the voice wants/thinks/feels), agency (the voice will 'make something happen'), or identity (the voice 'comes' from somewhere or has a specific and idiosyncratic ontological status). Complexity ... will typically involve a voice being attributed multiple, qualitatively different person-like states. (Alderson-Day et al., 2021: 233)

Based on these definitions, the CASS research team drew on concepts from literary linguistic theory to develop a characterisation model through which analysts could formalise the documentation of personness in the descriptions of voices by voice-hearers (see Semino et al., 2021).

In this chapter, we focus specifically on agency as a component of the HtV team's definitions for personification and our own view of recording personness (Semino et al., 2021). Agency has also been shown to be a key part of other taxonomies developed among clinical psychologists for describing personification (see Wilkinson and Bell, 2016). From a linguistic perspective, the CASS team was interested in a semantic view that allowed them to discuss *degrees* of agency, as opposed to a strictly binary grammatical view (i.e., who is active and who is passive in a clausal structure; Darics and Koller, 2019). As Darics and Koller (2019: 219) argue, 'Clearly, it is more agentive to effect a material change in the world ... than to merely become or be something'. To this end, we can refer to the transitivity model and the classification of process types to help us discuss the different ways in which social actors are reported to have agency.

10.3.2 Transitivity

Transitivity is one element of the complex system of linguistic analysis known as systemic functional linguistics (SFL), most commonly associated with Halliday (e.g., Halliday, 1994; Halliday and Matthiessen, 2014). Transitivity is oriented around meaning insofar as it represents the happenings around us, the states of affairs of the world, and our responses to them. The transitivity framework gives us the resources to describe and evaluate this flow of events 'as a configuration of elements centred on a process' (Halliday and Matthiessen, 2014: 213). These processes involve participants (who enact and are affected by these processes) and circumstances (how, when, and where these processes occur). Each component can broadly be mapped onto clausal elements – that is, the participants are typically realised in the nominal group (*it, the voices*), circumstances by the adverbial group (*today*) or prepositional phrase (*from next door*), and processes in the verbal group (*started, will be going*).

The various processes through which we can refer to the many different aspects of our experience have been classified into the following process types (Halliday and Matthiessen, 2014: 214–15):

- Material: construing the outer experience of physical actions
- Mental: representing the inner experience of thoughts and emotions
- Relational: referring to processes of identifying and classifying

- Behavioural: representing the outer manifestations of inner workings such as laughing or sleeping
- Verbal: concerned with saying and expressing meaning
- Existential: recognising the existence or happening of various phenomena

However, Halliday and Matthiessen (2014: 218) acknowledge that these are 'fuzzy categories'; in other words, the boundaries between them are not clear-cut. In response to ambiguities in the classification, alternative taxonomies have been developed and the prevailing schools in this area are those derived from Halliday (1994), known as the Sydney model (SM) and the Cardiff grammar (CG) model, best described in Fawcett (2000) and Neale (2002). The CG model proposes an alternative taxonomy for process types, namely action, mental, relational, influential, environmental, and event-relating. One of the key differences between the models is indicated in the influential category, which captures verbs such *start, try, continue,* or *stop,* as well as verbs that denote success and failure (Bartley, 2018). In our discussion, we will take the SM taxonomy as our starting point and refer to pertinent aspects of the CG model as they correspond with the challenges identified through the CASS research team's investigation of processes described in their interviews with voice-hearers.

10.3.3 Querying References to Voices

Since the CASS team were interested in the variety of labelling terms used to refer to voices, a preliminary task in their analysis was to locate references to voices in the participant responses. A member of the research team read through the interview transcripts and manually tagged references to voices in the corresponding corpus files. This process demonstrated how identifying a referent is based on contextual information, particularly in the case of pronouns (i.e., differentiating when 'it' referred to a voice and when it did not) and when the referent is introduced in a preceding turn. For example,

> Interviewer: you mentioned that two are male and one was female
> Participant: Female, yeah.

Manual identification of references to voices confirmed that the range of terms used was beyond the team's introspection and showed that voices could be invoked according to different parts of speech:

- Pronouns: *it, she, they*
- Nouns: *voices, shadow, Roxy*
- Determiners: *this, some, which*
- Verbs as gerunds: *commenting, whispering*
- Adjectives: for example, 'there's one *good* and one *bad*'

As such, the procedure of identifying references to voices in the first instance was not amenable to (a simple) corpus query. However, once the researchers had manually tagged references to voices in the data, they were able to run corpus queries for frequency and distribution of voice label types (see Collins et al., 2023). This allowed them to determine that there were 9,030 instances of references to voices in the data, expressed as 392 different types. The most common types were *it* (1952), *they* (1518), *he* (732), *she* (673), *them* (481), and *voices* (383).

Furthermore, the tagging of voice referents allowed the CASS team to perform additional queries that highlighted associated qualities and actions through adjective and verb collocates. In particular, the voice labels (i.e., the referents that we tagged) and their collocates directed the researchers to identification strategies that correspond with Van Leeuwen's (2008) social actor network. For example,

- Classification: *girl, man, feminine, childlike, old*
- Relational: *dad, ex-girlfriend*
- Physical: *big, angular*
- Appraisement: *evil, clever, useless*

These are discussed in some detail by Collins and colleagues (2023), including which kinds of labelling strategies are favoured in cases of minimal and/or complex personification. Here, we consider the reporting of actions, positing the voices as social actors with various degrees of agency.

10.3.4 Classifying Process Types

The investigation of processes associated with voices was guided by the identification of verb collocates of the voice labels that the researchers tagged. The proximity of a referent and a verb does not entail a definite clausal relationship (i.e., we cannot assume that the verb is carried out by or acts upon our node as a participant in the clause). Nevertheless, we can set our collocational window to maximally target subject-verb combinations. Manual checking of the outputs from alternative settings (i.e., three/four/five tokens to the left/right of the node) showed that three tokens to the right of the node were optimal for the precision and recall of processes directly attributable to a voice. The research team set a minimum frequency of one as an association measure in order to capture the full list of verb collocates. They identified 462 different lemmatised verb types, the most common of which were *be* (1569), *say* (433), *come* (280), *go* (270), *do* (265), *get* (252), and *tell* (230).

The researchers then considered automatically categorising the verb collocate types according to Halliday and Matthiessen's (2014) taxonomy; in other words, collating the verb types that correspond with each process type category

10.3 Investigating the Agency of Voices in Psychosis

(*talk* as verbal; *think* as mental, etc.). However, it was problematic to reduce each verb type to a singular meaning that corresponded with just one process type category. Other researchers have found that because it is a semantically oriented task, there is a range of contextual factors, along with different usage patterns, that make it difficult to develop algorithms for automatic process-type classification (Yan, 2014). As such, while the CASS team's observations began with a table of the verb collocates and their frequency, the researchers' interpretations were based on instances as they occurred in the original context of the interview.

One of the first steps in classifying process types is to identify the main process in a clause. Bartley (2018: 12) explains that there are differences in how the SM and CG model instruct analysts to approach phrasal elements with a catenative verb. These differences apply to verb phrases such as

- She *started talking* about them.
- He *wants to hurt* me.
- They're just *trying to distract* me.

In such cases, the SM would tend to focus on *talking*, *hurt* and *distract* as processes, whereas the CG model considers *started*, *wants* and *trying* to be the main processes. Furthermore, verbs such as *start* and *try* typify the influential process category in the CG model. Researchers must establish whether they will record one or both these elements of the process and decide which model they want to refer to, if they are looking to (quantitatively) describe patterns according to these top-level process types. Choosing either the SM or the CG model will generate very different views of the (same) data.

In the analysis of the voice-hearer interviews, while the researchers might collectively address the category 'material processes' based on the prevailing meaning of terms such as *control*, *fight*, and *hurt*, it is important to acknowledge the significance of the extended verbal group (*trying to hurt*), given its clear relevance to the discussion of capabilities and intentions – in other words, agency (see the definitions provided in Section 10.3.1). There are other instances in which the researchers focussed on the particular elements of a verbal phrase, based on its relevance to the inquiry into agency. For example, Collins and co-authors (2019: 48) discuss the qualitative differences in how verbs such as *stop* are used: the intransitive form (e.g., *the voices stopped*) demonstrates very limited agency; however, in the non-finite complementation clause 'they've *stopped me from doing* so much', the voice-hearer is explicitly attributing a negative outcome to the voice, which is shown to have the capacity to 'make something happen'.

The CASS research team found that the capacity of the voice(s) to communicate was of particular significance to their investigation, with communication verbs such as terms *say*, *tell*, and *talk* appearing as high-frequency collocates of references to voices. Bartley (2018: 13) is critical of the CG model for its classification of communicative processes (under the mental cognition category), as this seems to understate the significance of the action of deliberately transferring information to other sources – which has direct relevance to our discussion of the agency of voices. Verbal processes are treated as a distinct category in the SM and defined as covering 'any kind of symbolic exchange of meaning' (Halliday, 1994: 140). Among the terms that are included in this category, it is possible to further differentiate levels of agency and impact. For example, Collins and colleagues (2019: 48) discuss how *respond* and *answer* indicate the capacity for voice-hearers to participate in dialogue with their voices. This is particularly significant when the unidirectional nature of *threats* and *shouting* is often reported as a source of distress for voice-hearers, when they have limited options for affecting the interpersonal and communicative dynamic.

Similarly, there are certain mental processes that describe different levels of intent and subsequently – different degrees of surveillance or antagonism that can be a source of distress for voice-hearers. For instance, some voices are reported to *judge*, *embarrass*, *hate*, or *reassure* the voice-hearer, demonstrating their capacity to 'want/think/feel' (Alderson-Day et al., 2021). Bartley (2018: 5) explains that the subcategorisation of the CG model offers more detail – compared with the SM – for distinguishing 'the act of consciously perceiving something and doing so intuitively', which we can see in the comparison between *saw* versus *looked* and *hear* versus *listen*. This distinction can be particularly useful in capturing the perceived intent behind the voice *ignoring* the voice-hearer, for example.

10.3.5 Considerations for Investigating Transitivity

In this exploration of voice-hearer accounts, we have established that the concepts of agency and positing participants as social actors are of interest to researchers working in disciplines beyond linguistics, but that language-based theories offer frameworks for documenting dimensions of identification and agency in the labelling strategies and description of processes. While there are established frameworks that are predicated on shared principles for how agency is encoded in language, we have seen that there are different approaches to categorising processes. This means that researchers will need to critically reflect on which aspects they are particularly interested in capturing, particularly if they are looking to provide quantification, since fundamental steps such as identifying the main process in a clause will have implications for what is categorised and how. The different practices for documenting processes and related participants show how this is an analytical procedure that is difficult to automate; nevertheless, we have shown how wordlists and collocation analysis (following annotation) can help in identifying the most common terms used to denote participants and processes. Subsequently, we have considered some of the complexities in how processes are described. Given these complexities, processes that appear in the data warrant close, contextualised examination – particularly for the purposes of discerning degrees of agency attributed to different social actors in the text.

10.4 Conclusion

In this chapter we have demonstrated the value of investigating representations of social actors in two different health-related contexts. We have shown that documenting nomination strategies can involve different combinations of human introspection, corpus procedures such as generating wordlists and keywords, and outputs from large language model-based chatbot systems such as ChatGPT. Such combinations reiterate that while frequency-based approaches help establish prevailing patterns for language use, it is also useful to append these techniques with those that are less dependent on frequency, in order to try to capture the breadth of ways in which people talk about those experiencing various health challenges. Similarly, automated processes have their limitations in capturing the polysemy of lexical forms, and the human analyst has an important role to play, not only in choosing and implementing the framework for documenting social actors, but also in interpreting their position in the text and their reported contribution to wider social practices.

References

Alderson-Day, B., Woods, A., Moseley, P., Common, S., Deamer, F., Dodgson, G. and Fernyhough, C. (2021). Voice-Hearing and Personification: Characterizing Social Qualities of Auditory Verbal Hallucinations in Early Psychosis. *Schizophrenia Bulletin*, *47*(1), 228–36. https://doi.org/10.1093/schbul/sbaa095.

Baker, P., Gabrielatos, C. and McEnery. T. (2013). *Discourse Analysis and Media Attitudes: The Representation of Islam in the British Press*. Cambridge University Press.

Bartley, L. V. (2018). Putting Transitivity to the Test: A Review of the Sydney and Cardiff Models. *Functional Linguistics*, *5*(4), 1–21. https://doi.org/10.1186/s405 54-018-0056-x.

Brookes, G. and Baker, P. (2021) *Obesity in the News: Language and Representation in the Press*. Cambridge University Press.

Collins, L. C., Brezina, V., Demjén, Z., Semino, E. and Woods, A. (2023). Corpus Linguistics and Clinical Psychology: Investigating Personification in First-Person Accounts of Voice-Hearing. *International Journal of Corpus Linguistics*, *28*(1), 28–59. https://doi.org/10.1075/ijcl.21019.col.

Darics, E. and Koller, V. (2019). Social Actors "to Go": An Analytical Toolkit to Explore Agency in Business Discourse and Communication. *Business and*

Professional Communication Quarterly, *82*(2), 214–38. https://doi.org/10.1177/ 2329490619828367.

Fawcett, R. P. (2000). In Place of Halliday's Verbal Group Part 1: Evidence from the Problems of Halliday's Representations and the Relative Simplicity of the Proposed Alternative. *Word*, *51*(2), 157–203. https://doi.org/10.1080/ 00437956.2000.11432500.

Giddens, A. (1984). *The Constitution of Society: Outline of the Theory of Structuration*. Polity Press.

Halliday, M. A. K. (1994). *An Introduction to Functional Grammar*, 2nd ed. Edward Arnold.

Halliday, M. A. K. and Matthiessen, C. (2014). *Halliday's Introduction to Functional Grammar*, 4th ed. Routledge.

Hardie, A. (2012). CQPweb: Combining Power, Flexibility and Usability in a Corpus Analysis Tool. *International Journal of Corpus Linguistics*, *17*(3), 380–409. https://doi.org/10.1075/ijcl.17.3.04har.

Lindenmayer, M. D. and Khan, A. (2006). Psychopathology. In J. A. Lieberman, T. S. Stroup and D. O. Perkins (eds.), *Textbook of Schizophrenia* (pp. 187–222). American Psychiatric Publishing. https://doi.org/10.1016/j.psc.2007.04.005.

Maller, C. J. (2015). Understanding Health through Social Practices: Performance and Materiality in Everyday Life. *Sociology of Health & Illness*, *37*(1), 52–66. https:// doi.org/10.1111/1467-9566.12178.

Neale, A. C. (2002). *More Delicate Transitivity: Extending the Process Type System Networks for English to Include Full Semantic Classifications*. Dissertation. Cardiff University. www.isfla.org/Systemics/Print/Theses/amy_neale_final_th esis.pdf.

Reisigl, M. and Wodak, R. (2001). *Discourse and Discrimination: Rhetorics of Racism and Antisemitism*. Routledge.

Semino, E., Demjén, Z. and Collins, L. (2021). Person-ness of Voices in Lived Experience Accounts of Psychosis: Combining Literary Linguistics and Clinical Psychology. *Medical Humanities*, *47*(3), 354–64. https://doi.org/10.1136/med hum-2020-011940.

Van Leeuwen, T. (1996). The Representation of Social Actors. In C. R. Caldas-Coulthard and M. Coulthard (eds.), *Texts and Practices: Readings in Critical Discourse Analysis* (pp. 32–70). Routledge. https://doi.org/10.4324/ 9780203431382.

Van Leeuwen, T. (2008). *Discourse and Practice: New Tools for Critical Analysis*. Oxford University Press. https://doi.org/10.1093/acprof:oso/9780195323306.001.0001.

Wilkinson, S. and Bell, V. (2016). The Representation of Agents in Auditory Verbal Hallucinations. *Mind & Language*, *31*(1), 104–26. https://doi.org/10.1111/ mila.12096.

Woods, A., Alderson-Day, B. and Fernyhough, C. (2022). Voices in Psychosis: Interdisciplinary Listening. In A. Woods, B. Alderson-Day and C. Fernyhough (eds.), *Voices in Psychosis: Interdisciplinary Perspectives* (pp. 3–16). Oxford University Press.

Yan, H. (2014). Automatic Labelling of Transitivity Functional Roles. *Journal of World Languages*, *1*(2), 157–70. https://doi.org/10.1080/21698252.2014.937563.

11 Positions Legitimated

11.1 Introduction

In this chapter we consider the phenomenon of legitimation. Legitimation can be considered as 'the process by which speakers accredit or license a type of social behavior'. Legitimation is enacted by argumentation – that is, through the provision of arguments 'that explain our social actions, ideas, thoughts, declarations, etc.' (Reyes, 2011: 782). One of the most common goals of legitimation in discourse, then, is to seek approval or acceptance from others, especially in cases where one might present a potentially controversial action as being an action which serves a wider group or community in some way.

Linguists and discourse analysts have established various frameworks for studying legitimation. Perhaps most notably, Van Leeuwen (2007; see also Van Leeuwen, 2008) identified four major categories of legitimation based on analysis of texts that were deemed to legitimate or de-legitimate compulsory education, such as children's books, brochures for parents, teacher training texts, and media texts. The categories of legitimation outlined by Van Leeuwen (2007: 92) were as follows:

- Authorization; that is, legitimation by reference to the authority of tradition, custom and law, and of persons in whom institutional authority of some kind is vested
- Moral evaluation; that is, legitimation by (often very oblique) reference to value systems
- Rationalization; that is, legitimation by reference to the goals and uses of institutionalised social action, and to the knowledge society has constructed to endow them with cognitive validity
- Mythopoesis; that is, legitimation conveyed through narratives whose outcomes reward legitimate actions and punish non-legitimate actions

Importantly, Van Leeuwen (2007) reiterates that strategies of legitimation can occur alone or in combination with each other within discourse. Central to the kinds of legitimation identified in the case studies to be discussed in this chapter is the notion of 'expertise'. We should thus note at this point that the first of these categories, 'Authorization', can be predicated on expert authority, in which case 'legitimacy is provided by expertise rather than status' (Van Leeuwen, 2007: 94). Significantly for many studies of health communication, including in the studies to be described in this chapter, this is distinct from authority granted by institutional status or customary tradition, for example, and can thus be invoked by social actors who might be less empowered than others in given health(care) settings, such as patients and practitioners.

In the sections that follow, we consider two case studies in which legitimation has been examined in the context of health communication, using corpus linguistic techniques. First, we describe research on legitimation in the context of disclosures of vaccine hesitancy. Second, we consider a study on patient feedback on healthcare services which considered, among other things, how patients contributing the feedback legitimated their comments and the evaluations of healthcare services and practitioners therein. Taken together, these case studies represent, respectively, a case in which legitimation in discourse was explicitly searched for and identified, and then a case in which legitimation was not expressly searched for but emerged as a discursive strategy within the data as part of a more general (corpus-based) discourse analysis.

11.2 Legitimation of Vaccine Hesitancy

In this section we show how corpus linguistic tools can be used to study how contributors to an online parenting forum legitimate their position in relation to the label 'anti-vaxxer', particularly by negating the applicability of that label to themselves (e.g., 'I am not an anti-vaxxer but . . . ').

As noted previously (see Section 3.3), the refusal or hesitancy to take up vaccinations for oneself or one's children has been labelled 'vaccine hesitancy' by the World Health Organization (WHO) and was included in 2019 among the top-10 global health threats. A 2014 WHO report from the Strategic Advisory Group of Experts on Immunization (SAGE) mentions three categories of determinants of vaccine hesitancy: (1) 'contextual influences' (e.g., religion, culture, politics, media environment); (2) individual and group influences (e.g., previous personal experiences with vaccinations, vaccination as a social norm or as not needed or harmful); and (3) vaccine/vaccination-specific issues (e.g., new vaccine, mode of administration, risks versus benefits).

More precisely, however, vaccine hesitancy tends to be described as a scale, involving different degrees and kinds of vaccination-related attitudes and behaviours (e.g., Larson et al., 2015). The label 'anti-vax' or 'anti-vaxxer' tends to be used informally – as well as in some published studies (e.g., Gravelle et al., 2022) – for the most vaccine-hesitant end of the scale.

Recent survey-based research has found, however, that a relatively small proportion of the population self-identifies as an 'anti-vaxxer' or can be appropriately described as such. Motta and co-authors (2023) report that out of 5,010 US-based respondents to a survey, 8 per cent fully identify with the anti-vaxxer label, while an additional 14 per cent say that they do so 'sometimes'. Motta's team also found that adopting an anti-vaxxer identity provides a potentially beneficial sense of belonging to a like-minded group which goes beyond the rejection of vaccines and particularly includes a distrust of scientific expertise. Gravelle and colleagues (2022) analysed 13,251 responses to a vaccination-related survey from the UK, the US, and Canada; based on a four-point scale of vaccine attitudes, they place in the 'anti-vax' group 3 per cent of UK respondents and 7 per cent of both US and Canadian respondents. However, they also note that 'a large percentage of the public in each country has mixed attitudes towards vaccines', while strong support is associated with older age, higher levels of education, and left-wing political views (Gravelle et al., 2022: 8).

Several typologies have been proposed of arguments against vaccinations, mainly based on the analysis of online interactions and anti-vaccination websites. In Table 11.1 and the following section, we draw from Fasce and colleagues' (2023) taxonomy, which is based on a systematic review of 152 scientific articles published between 1967 and 2021. Within this taxonomy, anti-vaccination arguments may draw from one or more of 62 themes, which are subsumed under 11 'attitude roots ... the psychological predispositions that lead people to selectively search for and adopt arguments to oppose vaccination' (Fasce et al., 2023: 1463).

Against this background, we have used a corpus that was created as part of the Questioning Vaccination Discourse project (Quo VaDis; www.lancaster.ac.uk/vaccination-discourse/) to study how contributors to the online parenting forum Mumsnet legitimate the statement that they are not 'anti-vax'.

11.2.1 Vaccine Hesitancy on Mumsnet

Founded in 2000, the parenting website Mumsnet reported 104 million unique user visits in 2019 and receives 1.2 billion page views per year (Mumsnet, 2021). Its forum section, Mumsnet Talk, currently hosts 243 topics via sub-forums organised around a specific subject, such as 'Children's health', 'Coronavirus', and 'Am I Being Unreasonable?' (AIBU). Vaccinations are one of the topics that contributors to Mumsnet write about. Indeed, a 2017 study found that 29 per cent of parents in England who use the internet as a source of vaccine-related information specifically access Mumsnet (Campbell et al., 2017).

As part of the Quo VaDis project, preliminary analysis of a corpus containing 895 threads of vaccination-related discussion, amounting to 6,269,560 words, attests to the prevalence of conflictual positions within family networks with respect to vaccination (reported in Coltman-Patel et al., 2022).

Table 11.1 *Fasce et al.'s (2023) taxonomy of anti-vaccination arguments*

Attitude roots	Themes
Conspiracy ideation	Government cover-up; Big pharma; Population control; Made-up threat; Targeting the disadvantaged
Distrust	Negligent healthcare; Untrustworthy data; It is just a theory; Exaggerated risk; Financial interests; Systemic corruption; Absence of liability; Oppressive outgroups; Do your own research
Unwarranted beliefs	Alternative medicine; Natural is best; Overmedicalization; Alternatives to vaccination; Science denial; Absurd causality; Vaccinated are a threat; Fallacious logic; Disease disappears by itself
Worldview and politics	Science-related populism; Libertarianism; Politicization of vaccines; Traditionalism; Rejection of modernity
Religious concerns	Impurity; Appeal to natural order; Religious authority; The work of God; Religious exemptions
Moral concerns	Unethical experimentation; Anti-abortion position; Sexual promiscuity; Health is not business; Anti-utilitarianism; Bad parenting
Fears and phobias	Side effects; Safety concerns; Dreadful injuries; Toxicity hazard; Contraindications; Immune compromise; Trypanophobia
Distorted risk perception	Vaccination is unnecessary; Disease is not serious; Misperception of risk; Cost-benefit analysis; Vaccination is not for me
Perceived self-interest	Free-riding; Luxury measures
Epistemic relativism	Truth is relative; Anecdotal evidence; Epistemic superiority; Individualistic epistemology; All or nothing
Reactance	Resisting coercion; Personal autonomy; Vindication of civil liberties; Going against the herd

From Fasce et al., 2023: 1468–9.

Furthermore, the analysis demonstrates the presence of a negative, sometimes antagonistic, attitude towards people who may be perceived as 'anti-vaxxers'. For example,

> Unless there is a known family history of certain allergies the case against vaccination is a load of dangerous hippy bullshit. Yes there have been some cases of vaccinations causing harm but this is shit bad luck the same as if your beloved child gets leukaemia or is hit by a bus.

Despite the contributor's dismissive attitude towards the position of being 'against' vaccination, there is an appeal to rationality ('unless there is a known family history') and some mitigation on the basis that certain circumstances might justify 'vaccine hesitancy' (i.e., the risk of harm).

In view of this, we report on a small study of the expression and qualification of ideological positions in relation to vaccinations. In what follows, we will focus on contributions to the forum in which individuals dissociate from the identity of

11.2 Legitimation of Vaccine Hesitancy

'anti-vaxxer' (i.e., someone who is ideologically opposed to vaccination). However, what we will show is that this tends to indicate a more complex and considered position, whereby participants take 'anti-vaccination' as a point of reference but explain that the position is insufficient or undesirable in some way that precludes them from adopting the identity unreservedly. Thus, in establishing an 'anti-vaccination' position as the nexus, the contributor creates a point of comparison for their own ideas, which are variously likened or contrasted with the notions associated with 'anti-vaccination'.

Our analysis is conducted using the Quo VaDis Mumsnet corpus: 31,211,157 words consisting of 12,288 threads from 41 Mumsnet Talk topics with Original posts containing the strings 'vac*', 'vaxx*', or 'jab*' (where the asterisk stands for zero or any character or a sequence of characters), with optional prefixes un (-), re(-), anti(-), and pro(-).

11.2.2 Identifying Ideological Positions about Vaccination

We set out to retrieve from the Mumsnet corpus expressions of self-reference in relation to vaccination – that is, occurrences of the first-person singular pronoun *I* in close proximity to mentions of vaccines or vaccinations. To that end, we established the query I ++* (*vac*|*vax*); this query syntax allowed for variation in the syntactical relationship and premodification of the reference to the vaccine (indicated in the ++* component), as well as variation in the lexical form of reference to the vaccine/vaccination, as indicated in the (*vac*|*vax*) component. The query returned 11,370 matches in 3,203 different texts and generated a list of 5,306 different formulations, the most frequent of which (30+ occurrences) are shown in Table 11.2.

The research team was not interested in reports of people having a vaccination, nor their intention to do so, but rather contributors' positioning of themselves in relation to labels suggesting attitudes towards vaccinations, such as 'pro-vaccine' and 'anti-vax'. While participants appeared to claim a 'pro-vaccination' stance for themselves ('I'm very pro vaccine'), references to an 'anti-vax' position were more commonly dissociative, as in 'I'm not an antivaxxer'. This can be expected, given the evidence that in these Mumsnet discussions, pro-vaccination contributors sometimes respond rather aggressively to views and behaviours that may be described as anti-vaccination (Coltman-Patel et al., 2022). Subsequently, we refined our query to target self-references in relation to an 'anti-vaccination' perspective, as follows: I ++* (anti-va*|antiva*|anti va*) for further investigation. This query generated 1,093 occurrences from 480 different texts, which were expressed according to 457 different formulations. The most common are shown in Table 11.3.

Table 11.2 *Most frequent formulations resulting from the query I ++* (*vac*|*vax*)*

Rank	Phrase	Occurrences
1	I had the vaccine	379
2	I had my vaccine	175
3	I've had the vaccine	154
4	I've been vaccinated	128
5	I had the AZ vaccine	125
6	I think the vaccine	99
7	i wasn't vaccinated	83
8	I'm not anti vax	72
9	I got the vaccine	67
10	i have been vaccinated	64
11	I didn't vaccinate	61
12	I had my first vaccine	61
13	I have had the vaccine	59
14	I had the pfizer vaccine	56
15	I am pro vaccine	55
16	I'm not an anti-vaxxer	53
17	I'm not anti-vax	53
18	I'm pro vaccine	49
19	I've had my vaccine	48
20	I will have the vaccine	48
21	I'm fully vaccinated	46
22	I get the vaccine	46
23	I have the vaccine	46
24	I had my vaccination	44
25	I am pro vaccination	42
26	I'm not anti vaccine	39
27	I would have the vaccine	39
28	I don't vaccinate	38
29	I had the vaccination	37
30	I'm very pro vaccine	34
31	I had the oxford vaccine	33
32	I want the vaccine	33
33	I wouldn't vaccinate	33
34	I haven't vaccinated	31
35	I'm a vaccinator	30
36	I am not anti vax	30
37	I had been vaccinated	30

The next step of the analysis was to examine concordance lines and determine how the referent of the 'anti-va*|antiva*|anti va*' label indicated an ideological position.

11.2 Legitimation of Vaccine Hesitancy

Table 11.3 *Most frequent formulations resulting from the query I++* (anti-va*|antiva*|anti va*)*

Rank	Phrase	Occurrences
1	I'm not anti vax	72
2	I'm not an anti vaxxer	56
3	I'm not an anti-vaxxer	53
4	I'm not anti-vax	53
5	I'm not anti vaccine	39
6	I am not anti vax	30
7	I'm not anti vaccination	23
8	I'm not anti-vaccine	22
9	I am not anti vaccine	22
10	I am not an anti Vaxxer	20
11	I am not anti-vaccine	20
12	I am not an anti-vaxxer	17
13	I am not anti vaccination	14
14	I am not anti-vax	14
15	I'm not anti-vaccination	13
16	I'm not an anti vaxer	11

11.2.3 Discursive Strategies for Legitimating Vaccine Hesitancy

The first step in our analysis was to separate those occurrences that referred to a third party, rather than the contributor themselves (e.g., 'I have friends who are anti-vax', 'I have not seen any anti-vaxx posts'). Of the 1,093 occurrences returned from our query, 284 (25.98 per cent) actually refer to someone or something else. What remained were 809 (74.02 per cent) occurrences in which participants describe their own ideological position in relation to an 'anti-vaccination' perspective. We observed only 6 (0.55 per cent) instances in which contributors claimed an anti-vaccination perspective for themselves:

> Yes i am proudly antivax and have been for a few years now. (Discussion topic: General health)

For the most part, contributors referred to how their beliefs misalign with what they recognise to be 'anti-vax', which involved various degrees of dissociation or qualification. For example, in the following extract the author disassociates themselves unequivocally from the *anti-vaxxer* label:

> I'm not an anti-vaxxer in the slightest, and I despair at those who are. (AIBU)

In contrast, the author of the next extract qualifies their position in relation to the label:

> I'm not completely anti vaccination but we have a strong family history of allergy/asthma etc so have to weigh that up (General health)

Several contributors problematise the absolute position of 'anti-vaxxer' and state that the label is used to dismiss and distance people who express anything other than complete support for vaccines and vaccination schedules:

> I'm not an anti-vaxxer either though – it's just an accusation that gets thrown at anyone on MN who has any questions/concerns about vaccines/delays vaccines/ selectively vaccinates or has any issue with any vaccine or its timing in the UK vaccine schedule tbh. (AIBU)

Furthermore, while the 'anti-vaxxer' label is often posited in binary opposition to the 'pro-vaccination' label, some posters offer the alternative stance of being 'pro-choice' – an argument that Fasce and co-authors (2023) capture via the 'Personal autonomy' theme:

> I'm not an anti-vaxxer. My family are all up to date with vaccinations. I am pro choice (Behaviour development)

In the previous example, the statement that the writer's family 'are all up to date with vaccinations' is used to establish their credentials as someone who is not anti-vaccination. In our data, the provision of this kind of detail often occurs in close proximity to the negation of the anti-vaxxer identity.

In several instances, contributors negotiate additional positions of vaccine hesitancy along a cline by presenting anti-vax as a matter of degree, as suggested by the expressions 'I'm not completely anti-vaccination', 'I'm not particularly anti-vaccine', or 'I am more anti-vaccine than pro-vaccine'. In most cases, however, rather than alluding to a scale of attitudes towards vaccinations, contributors set out to legitimate their position by making explicit in what specific respect they may adopt a critical position towards vaccinations or not take a particular vaccination.

The most commonly cited concern expressed in the data relates to the (potential) harmful effects of the vaccine. This tends to involve arguments that Fasce and colleagues (2023) capture via the themes relating to the 'Fears and phobias' attitude root, such as 'Safety concerns' and 'Dreadful injuries'. In many cases, such concerns were informed by personal or family circumstances of medical histories, reflecting the individual dimension in SAGE's (2014) categorisation of determinants of vaccine hesitancy:

> I'm not an anti-vax person at all! Just having lost a baby before and having severe anxiety and depression during this pregnancy it's not an easy thing to do hence the fact I've left it so long (Pregnancy)

> Thanks but DS can't have it. The last vaccine he had nearly killed him (no I'm not an anti-vaxxer – [his temperature shot up, wouldn't come down despite plying him with copious amounts of Calpol and nurofen] and he ended up in hospital with major breathing problems) (AIBU)

11.2 Legitimation of Vaccine Hesitancy

The provision of details about serious health-related events arguably involves the legitimation strategy of rationalization, in that each writer has very good reasons for their concerns about vaccinations. At the same time, the disclosure of traumatic personal circumstances also appeals to emotion. The first example also explicitly references the writer's emotional state following the trauma of losing a baby ('severe anxiety and depression'). Furthermore, we also find examples of mini narratives that serve as cautionary tales and demonstrate Van Leeuwen's (2007) category of mythopoesis.

Relatedly, the novelty of the vaccines is one of the factors leading to speculation about their potentially harmful effects. The 2014 WHO report noted previously mentions specifically the introduction of new vaccines as one of the causes of this kind of vaccine hesitancy (SAGE, 2014: 12). In our data, the strategy for redirecting efforts towards swift development of the vaccines against COVID-19 – in particular – introduced doubt as to whether they had undergone sufficient testing in the first place, alongside concerns regarding the as-yet unknown long-term effects:

> I am not a fan of rushed-through vaccines, there needs to be proper testing. There's no way I would have such a vaccine, and I'm not an anti-vaxxer. (Coronavirus)

> I'm not an anti-vaxxer, my son has had his vaccines. I'm just wary of new vaccines for historical reasons: www.ncbi.nlm.nih.gov/pmc/articles/PMC1383764/ (Coronavirus)

> No I won't be getting it immediately, we've all had our jabs so I'm not an anti-vaxxer by any means. I feel it's too rushed and the long term side affects aren't known yet (Coronavirus)

The previous examples are typical of our data from the 'Coronavirus' topic on Mumsnet in that they all mention previous vaccinations as part of the writer's credentials as a non-anti-vaxxer. They include different strategies for authorisation (the hyperlink to a scientific paper in the first example) and rationalisation (through references to what is 'known').

A very specific approach to the presentation of oneself as a rational agent capable of making decisions involves referencing one's own 'research' (see also the previous discussion on 'informed', and Fasce et al.'s (2023) 'Do your own research' theme):

> I am not an anti-vacs person but I do like to research the decisions I make for my family (Pregnancy)

This implicitly suggests a lack of trust in how scientific findings are used in vaccination programmes and policies, as well as a belief in one's own ability to acquire sufficient expertise to make independent decisions.

The importance of autonomy and independent decision-making is also reflected in the major theme of resisting mandated vaccination. Some writers express disagreement with vaccination-related policies, the coverage of the vaccination programme, or elements of compulsion (see Fasce et al.'s (2023) 'Resisting coercion' theme):

> I'm really not anti-vax in any way. I volunteered for the coronavirus vaccine trials and will have the vaccine when available. I just don't personally agree with compulsory vaccinations. (Coronavirus)

> I am not anti-vaccine I am anti a vaccination policy that demands that everyone aim at herd immunity regardless of their childs history and vulnerability. (Children's health)

Others make a distinction between 'necessary' and, by implication, unnecessary vaccinations, and claim to take up only the former:

> I am not anti vaccinations at all but I do like to know that they are necessary before I have them or allow my children to have them. (AIBU)

> No way am I taking two doses of a vaccine I don't need and I'm not an antivaccer (AIBU)

In all these cases, the legitimation of the writer's position relies primarily on their rational ability to assess policy and the necessity of vaccinations on a case-by-case basis. The rejection of mandatory vaccinations also potentially involves moral evaluation, insofar as the writer is concerned about the implications of compulsion for fellow citizens.

Lack of trust is more explicitly present when references are made to the unreliability of governments and pharmaceutical companies:

> I'm not an anti-vaxxer at all, but I don't understand why people suddenly seem to blindly trust our corrupt government and these terrible drug companies to have out best interests at heart, when time and time again they've shown that they don't. (Coronavirus)

> I am not anti vaccines- myself and my family are up to date with our vaccines but I do question the government's desperation and I wonder why others follow blindly what the government is feeding them. (Coronavirus)

This kind of argument is captured by Fasce's team (2023) in the themes 'Government cover-up' and 'Big Pharma' (from the 'Conspiracy ideation' attitude root) and is included under 'contextual influences' in SAGE's (2014) report. In our examples, a position of mistrust is presented as different and separate from being an anti-vaxxer. The first example also makes explicit how the writer sees trust as less rational than the position they have adopted (cf. 'blindly trust').

Finally, a frequent qualification of the writer's position in relation to vaccination involves the rejection of specific vaccines, or combinations of vaccines, reflecting SAGE's 'vaccine/vaccination-specific issues' as a major determinant of vaccine hesitancy:

I'm not an anti-vaxxer at all, me and my kids have had all other jabs, but I'm not convinced with this one. [flu vaccine] (Pregnancy)

I'm not an anti-vaxxer and modern medicine has saved my life on more than one occasion. However, I question the wisdom of overloading little immune systems with up to 19 vaccines in one go, I think it should be spread across several injections over the months. (AIBU)

Such contributions challenge the wholesale adoption of an 'anti-vaxx' philosophy in arguing for the assessment of each vaccine according to its individual merits. The final example reflects a common concern surrounding the number of vaccines that are administered, particularly when seen in relation to the perceived vulnerability of infants.

In summary, the principled selection of concordance lines involving the firstperson negation of an anti-vaxxer identity has led us to identify the range of ways in which Mumsnet contributors reject that identity while at the same time legitimating a nuanced position in relation to vaccinations. By and large, this involves the use of Van Leeuwen's (2007) legitimation strategy of rationalization – that is, the process of legitimating a position by referring to knowledge and the cognitive validity of positions presented as reasonable, acceptable, appropriate, or even superior to those who may disagree. On the one hand, our observations are consistent with previous findings that the identity of 'anti-vaxxer' is adopted by a relatively small proportion of people, while a much larger proportion have some specific concerns about vaccinations that coexist with taking up available vaccines most of the time. On the other hand, we have shown how the concerns and qualifications that are presented in our data as consistent with *not* being an anti-vaxxer are captured by existing typologies of determinants of vaccine hesitancy and well-known arguments against vaccination.

11.3 Legitimation of Patient Evaluations of Healthcare Services

In this section, we turn to a case study in which legitimation was identified as a recurring discursive strategy in corpus data, even though it was not explicitly searched for from the outset of the analysis. This work comes from the wider programme of research on patient feedback introduced in Chapter 6. In that chapter, we saw how, faced with the absence of reliable demographic metadata, the researchers involved in that project had to rely on patients' disclosures of aspects of their identities within the comments themselves as a way of examining the possible influence of such identity factors on the feedback given (see Baker et al., 2019; Section 6.2 in this book). While this was an area of focus that was pursued in line with the questions set out by the healthcare provider partner on the project, the NHS, the resultant analyses indicated legitimation as a recurrent discursive strategy in the comments.

11.3.1 Strategies of Legitimation

One such example arose in the analysis of patients' comments that mentioned age. Specifically, it was found that (particularly older) patients frequently referred to their older age as part of a broader description of their experience using healthcare services. In such cases, Baker and colleagues (2019) argue, patients can index their experience as healthcare consumers and, accordingly, construct themselves as 'informed' or 'expert' patients (Fox et al., 2005), in this case as expert healthcare service users, in particular regarding regular standards of healthcare service provision and, as such, what they might reasonably expect. In this way, the patients positioned themselves as having reasonable expectations, thus rendering them as qualified and reasonable evaluators of the services they accessed. As detailed in Chapter 6, such comments were accessed through concordance searches of queries which were determined to be productive for identifying cases in which patients described their age (as opposed to, say, someone else's age or simply the number of years that they had been seeing a provider).

Such cases could indicate the legitimation of positive feedback. For example, in the following comment, a patient notes his age ('I am a 55 year old man') before then describing how he has 'been a patient with this surgery all my life'. This autobiographical segment was then followed by a positive appraisal of the practice, where the preceding segment served to legitimate this man's perspective as an experienced patient at the practice, with his evaluations being based not on a single visit but on consistently positive experiences over a long period of time ('I have always had a positive relationship with ... ').

> Caring, Supportive & Helpful GP & GP practice I am a 55 year old man, I have been a patient with this surgery all my life. I have always had a positive relationship with the Doctors, Nurses & Staff at [Anonymised] Medical practice.

However, this kind of self-construction of an experienced, 'expert' patient identity could also be used to legitimate negative feedback. This accords with Reyes's (2011) observation that legitimation strategies are typically invoked in order to justify contentious propositions. Indeed, negative feedback could be viewed as contentious – face-threatening, even (Austin, 1962) – when we bear in mind that such comments are directed at the providers themselves. For example, the following comment represents something of an inverse of that seen above. This patient described himself as 'over 60 years old with a lot of excellent dental practice on my teeth' before then providing a negative appraisal of the dental practice in question. This autobiographical segment serves two functions: in addition to (self-)constructing the commenter as an

11.3 Legitimation of Patient Evaluations of Healthcare Services

experienced, 'expert' patient, the evaluation of their past experiences as 'excellent' simultaneously presents them as a reasonable and balanced judge of such services, capable of praising services when they are good and criticising them when they are not. This latter point arguably takes on more pronounced importance in the context of particularly severe criticism; indeed, in the following comment, the patient describes the practice as 'by far the wors[t]' they have encountered, notes how they are 'still in a great deal of pain', and accuses the dentist of being 'oblivious to the challenges' that are particular to older patients' dental treatment requirements.

> I am over 60 years old with a lot of excellent dental practice on my teeth... and this is by far the worse I have ever encountered having moved to Chelmsford within the last year ... since the appointment ... I have still a great deal of pain ... the dentist seem oblivious to the challenges they have in regard to mature teeth of the older generation.

Additionally invoking what Van Leeuwen (2007) terms 'authorization' by describing their experience (and thereby indexing a kind of 'expertise') in their comments, some patients were also found to deploy argumentation based on 'moral evaluation' (Van Leeuwen, 2007) as means of legitimating their evaluations. As a reminder, moral evaluation is legitimation by (often very oblique) reference to value systems. As an example, the patient writing the following comment constructs himself as not being burdensome to the NHS, which keys into a moral discourse that public health systems should be used only when necessary (Llanwarne et al., 2017). The patient evokes this discourse by first noting his age ('73 year old male') and history of 'heart problems', which might set up an expectation that this patient has complex healthcare needs and would thus have to use the NHS frequently. However, the patient then describes how he consciously does not use the NHS very often, as he is aware of the strain that services are under ('tended not to visit my GP because I know they are very busy'). Moreover, when he uses such services, he does so rarely, only for routine appointments, and notes how he always attends these ('I only have a check up once a year which I always attend'), perhaps indicating an awareness of how much missed appointments cost the NHS (Llanwarne et al., 2017). We can also note how, at the end of the comment, the patient describes how 'considering going to A&E ... is totally against [his] principles', explicitly invoking a moral evaluation to again position himself as a conscientious user of healthcare services who is opposed to using Accident and Emergency services for non-emergencies and is aware of the issues that doing so would cause for the NHS (see, for example, Adamson et al., 2009). This background information helps establish this patient's credentials as a genuine and conscientious patient (as opposed to being a 'time-waster'), which then legitimates his complaint about a lack of appointment availability.

182 11 Positions Legitimated

> I am a 73 year old male with a history of heart problems but have in the past few years tended not to visit my GP because I know they are very busy and I only have a check up once a year which I always attend. If I have any minor ailments I tend to consult my local Chemist for advice. I had cause to visit my GP today 25/03/2015 to make an appointment, only to be told that the earliest appointment is in 13 days time on Tues. 07/04/2015. I was not even offered an appointment to see another GP in the Practice. This is an absolute disgrace and I am considering going to A&E. which is totally against my principles.

Another area in which patients appealed to value systems to legitimate their evaluations was with respect to ideas and attitudes relating to gender, specifically in the analysis of comments in which patients disclosed their identities as men or women. For example, in the following excerpt, a patient complains about the pain he experienced when having a filling put in at the dentist. He legitimates his account of the amount of pain he experienced by referring to the fact he is a 'a big 6ft man'. It is implied here that this patient would ordinarily be able to withstand a large amount of pain, and thus the pain that he experienced was exceptionally severe, prompting his complaint.

> Now I am a big 6ft man who has under gone a lot of dental work and have never felt pain like it. I ended up shaking and crying. I had to wait for an hour afterwards as I couldn't drive my car.

There were also cases of women mentioning their identities for similar reasons, for example, describing their pain threshold as high by referencing how many times they had given birth or describing how they had given birth with little or no pain relief, as in the following extract.

> I am not a soft woman I gave birth with no pain relief, that was an absolute doddle compared to this!

Overall, then, although Baker and colleagues (2019) did not explicitly set out to identify instances of legitimation strategies being used in the discourse of the patients' feedback, their qualitative examination of the comments revealed the recurring use of such strategies to contextualise – and, in the process, legitimate – the appraisals of healthcare services given. Such strategies were particularly visible in comments in which patients disclosed aspects of their identities (namely their age and sex identities). Where comments disclosing age tended to invoke a version of 'authorization' based on patients' implicit self-constructions of themselves as expert users of healthcare services, comments mentioning patients' sex identities tended to draw on moral values to construe patients as having a high threshold for pain tolerance. While legitimation strategies in age-based comments could be used to justify positive or negative feedback, those found in the gender-based comments tended to be used in support of negative appraisals. Baker and colleagues (2019) argue that the use of such legitimation strategies, particularly in the case of negative comments, could represent a means by which patients try to ensure that their comments and feedback will be taken seriously.

11.4 Conclusion

In this chapter, we have explored the ways in which corpus linguistic techniques can support the analysis of legitimation in health-related discourse. Through detailed case studies – ranging from analyses of vaccine hesitancy discussions on online forums, to patient evaluations of healthcare services – our exploration has highlighted the complex interplay of personal narratives, societal expectations, and medical authority in shaping public perceptions and behaviours with regard to health and health(care).

The examination of vaccine hesitancy on Mumsnet revealed not only the depth of personal conviction but also the societal and ideological undercurrents that influence such stances. Here, legitimation strategies are often deployed as part of a nuanced negotiation of identity, wherein individuals articulate their positions in relation to broader societal labels, such as 'anti-vaxxer', both to align themselves with but also distance themselves from charged public dialogue around this issue. Patient feedback on healthcare services, meanwhile, also offers a rich ground for observing legitimation in action. The patients analysed by Baker and colleagues (2019) were found to draw upon their personal experiences and societal roles – underscored by their age and/or gender identities – in order to lend credibility to their evaluations of healthcare services and healthcare providers. This act of self-positioning serves to authorise the patients' perspectives, potentially with the aim of ensuring that their comments will be valued and taken seriously by providers, particularly in cases in which comments expressed severe criticism.

These examples illustrate the role that corpus linguistic methods can play, then, in identifying and illuminating strategies of legitimation that are employed within different genres of health-related discourse. Notably, taken together, the case studies presented also showcase the versatility of corpus linguistic techniques in this endeavour. More specifically, while in the first case study legitimation strategies were searched for – perhaps in a fashion redolent of 'corpus-based' approaches – in the latter case study they were not expressly sought but emerged from the analysis, in a fashion we might associate more with 'corpus-driven' approaches. However legitimation might be approached, crucial to both approaches for the identification and analysis of legitimation strategies was the qualitative analysis of extended (and, as far as possible, contextualised) samples of the corpus data (or, better still, the entire texts in question). Such qualitative engagement was beneficial not only for understanding the rhetorical effects of such legitimation strategies but, before that point, for actually *identifying* such strategies. This is because legitimation strategies are certainly not driven by 'form' but represent the kinds of discursive functions that are difficult – if not impossible – to identify through automated methods and/or by looking at decontextualised lists of (key)words, collocates, or clusters. Indeed, as noted, some categories of legitimation strategies, such as those assigned to 'moral evaluation', are marked in terms of their often-subtle textual manifestations (being 'often very oblique'). With this in mind, and as the case studies discussed in this chapter demonstrate, any analysis of legitimation strategies in a corpus will benefit from – and perhaps even depend on – close, qualitative examination of the data by the human analyst.

References

Adamson, J., Ben-Shlomo, Y., Chaturvedi, N. and Donovan, J. (2009). Exploring the Impact of Patient Views on 'Appropriate' Use of Services and Help Seeking: A Mixed Method Study. *British Journal of General Practice*, 59(564), e226–33. https://doi.org/10.3399/bjgp09X453530.

Austin, J. L. (1962). *How to Do Things with Words*. Oxford University Press. https://doi.org/10.1093/acprof:oso/9780198245537.001.0001.

Baker, P., Brookes, G. and Evans, C. (2019). *The Language of Patient Feedback: A Corpus Linguistic Study of Online Health Communication*. Routledge. https://doi.org/10.4324/9780429259265.

Campbell, H., Edwards, A., Letley, L., Bedford, H., Ramsay, M. and Yarwood, J. (2017). Changing Attitudes to Childhood Immunisation in English Parents. *Vaccine*, 35(22), 2979–85. https://doi.org/10.1016/j.vaccine.2017.03.089.

Coltman-Patel, T., Dance, W., Demjén, Z., Gatherer, D., Hardaker, C. and Semino, E. (2022). 'Am I Being Unreasonable to Vaccinate My Kids against My Ex's Wishes?' – A Corpus Linguistic Exploration of Conflict in Vaccination Discussions on Mumsnet Talk's AIBU Forum. *Discourse, Context & Media*, 48, 100624. https://doi.org/10.1016/j.dcm.2022.100624.

Fasce, A., Schmid, P., Holford, D. L., Bates, L., Gurevych, I. and Lewandowsky, S. (2023). A Taxonomy of Anti-Vaccination Arguments from a Systematic Literature Review and Text Modelling. *Nature Human Behaviour*, 7(9), 1462–80. https://doi.org/10.1038/s41562-023-01644-3.

Fox, N. J., Ward, K. J. and O'Rourke, A. J. (2005). The 'Expert Patient': Empowerment or Medical Dominance? The Case of Weight Loss, Pharmaceutical Drugs and the Internet. *Social Science and Medicine*, 60(6), 1299–1309. https://doi.org/10.1016/j.socscimed.2004.07.005.

Gravelle, T. B., Phillips, J. B., Reifler, J. and Scotto, T. J. (2022). Estimating the Size of 'Anti-vax' and Vaccine Hesitant Populations in the US, UK, and Canada: Comparative Latent Class Modeling of Vaccine Attitudes. *Human Vaccines & Immunotherapeutics*, 18(1), 2008214. https://doi.org/10.1080%2F21645515.2021.2008214.

Larson, H. J., Jarrett, C., Schulz, W. S., Chaudhuri, M., Zhou, Y., Dube, E., Schuster, M., MacDonald, N. E., Wilson, R. and SAGE Working Group on Vaccine Hesitancy.

(2015). Measuring Vaccine Hesitancy: The Development of a Survey Tool. *Vaccine*, *33*(34), 4165–75. https://doi.org/10.1016/j.vaccine.2015.04.037.

Llanwarne, N., Newbould, J., Burt, J., Campbell, J. L. and Roland, M. (2017). Wasting the Doctor's Time? A Video-Elicitation Interview Study with Patients in Primary Care. *Social Science & Medicine*, *176*, 113–22. https://doi.org/10.1016/j.socscimed.2017.01.025.

Motta, M., Callaghan, T., Sylvester, S. and Lunz-Trujilo, K. (2023). Identifying the Prevalence, Correlates, and Policy Consequences of Anti-Vaccine Social Identity. *Politics, Groups, and Identities*, *11*(1), 108–22. https://doi.org/10.1080/21565503.2021.1932528.

Mumsnet. (2021). Advertising with Mumsnet. Available at www.mumsnet.com/info/advertising. Accessed 29 March 2024.

Reyes, A. (2011). Strategies of Legitimization in Political Discourse: From Words to Actions. *Discourse & Society*, *22*(6), 781–807. https://doi.org/10.1177/0957926511419927.

SAGE Working Group on Vaccine Hesitancy. (2014). Report of the SAGE Working Group on Vaccine Hesitancy. Available from www.asset-scienceinsociety.eu/sites/default/files/sage_working_group_revised_report_vaccine_hesitancy.pdf. Accessed 29 March 2024.

Van Leeuwen, T. (2007). Legitimation in Discourse and Communication. *Discourse & Communication*, *1*(1), 91–112. https://doi.org/10.1177/1750481307071986.

(2008). *Discourse and Practice: New Tools for Critical Analysis*. Oxford University Press. https://doi.org/10.1093/acprof:oso/9780195323306.001.0001.

12 Dissemination

12.1 Introduction

In this penultimate chapter, we turn to the process of disseminating research findings of corpus research in health communication. Readers of this book are likely to have access to advice on publishing within their own discipline from other sources. Therefore, in this chapter we focus particularly on (1) academic dissemination outside our own discipline, specifically in medical journals; (2) non-academic dissemination, including engagement with practitioners in healthcare, patient groups, and the media; and (3) potential evidence of influence on policy and practices (known as research 'impact' in the UK), and the difficulties of achieving and documenting such impact. The latter two aspects of doing research have increased in importance for the purposes of achieving funding in the UK and other countries over the last decade and are also the subject of debate (for linguistics, see McIntyre and Price, 2018, 2023; Mullany, 2020).

Here we will present two case studies. The first is concerned with the project on NHS feedback that we have already discussed in Chapters 2, 6, and 11. The second relates to the project on metaphors and cancer that we have already discussed in Chapters 5 and 9. One of the ways in which these two projects contrast is that the former was initiated by an approach from an external partner, and the researchers then worked with that partner all along (although not, as we will explain, with the same people). The latter project did not involve a single pre-established partner, but researchers worked both proactively and reactively to reach and interact with different potential groups of stakeholders. In both cases, what can be described as successful outcomes were achieved by facing partly unexpected challenges and taking up opportunities as they arose along the way.

12.2 Working with an External Partner: The NHS Feedback Project

This section is concerned with the experiences that two of the authors (Baker and Brookes) had when engaging with an external partner who had invited

12.2 Working with an External Partner

them to carry out work on data that the partners owned. In theory, dissemination in such a context ought to be relatively straightforward, as the researchers had been approached by the organisation, who clearly wanted them to analyse their data. However, we also discuss a number of complicating factors and unforeseen events which resulted in the engagement process being more challenging than expected.

12.2.1 Building Relationships and Achieving Impact

The project in question involved analysing a 40-million-word corpus of patient feedback and health practitioner responses that had been posted on a public NHS Choice website. A senior member of the Patients and Information Directorate at NHS England contacted the CASS research centre and asked if CASS members would be willing to carry out a corpus-assisted discourse analysis of the dataset, setting the researchers 12 questions (described in Section 2.4). The team was able to obtain funding from the ESRC to employ a full-time researcher for 18 months to assist with the analysis. During the project, there were regular meetings between CASS and members of the NHS England team, where the CASS team reported their findings and demonstrated the methodological techniques that they had used on the corpus.

There was a delay of several months between the first contact with NHS England and the point at which the analysis could begin. This delay was constituted by waiting for the funding application to the ESRC to be evaluated and processed, and then the period of advertising and appointing the research assistant. As a result, by the time that the researchers were ready to start the project, the contact person at NHS England had moved on to another post within the organisation. Additionally, the name of the team who dealt with NHS feedback had been changed. This meant that the researchers at CASS started the project with an unfamiliar contact person who did not know much about corpus linguistics or the reputation of the research centre. In large organisations, this kind of 'churn' is common, due to people seeking promotion or moving to and from other organisations. Thus, this is something to bear in mind when working with external partners. The researchers had to establish a relationship with a newly appointed contact person, and this meant that early meetings involved explaining their methodological approach to an extent that had not been anticipated.

Towards the end of the 18-month lifetime of the project, the new contact person also moved to a different position, so the researchers were assigned a third person to report to. It was fortunate that with both of these changes, the new contact person was open to working with CASS, and the third contact person arranged for the researchers to work on a second dataset, which involved feedback relating to cancer care (see Chapter 6). Therefore, it was felt that despite the changing nature of the organisation, it was possible to keep up a good relationship with key different individual members.

Not every NHS England staff member viewed the involvement of CASS as favourably, though. The researchers gave presentations at a range of NHS England meetings, with different people present, from different units. At one early meeting, the researchers spoke to a staff member who revealed that his unit had recently invested a large sum of money in a piece of software that was going to carry out all the analysis of NHS feedback without human intervention. When the researchers described the approach taken by CASS – using corpus software to identify the relevant aspects of the data, which would then need to be analysed and interpreted qualitatively by humans – the staff member made it clear he was not interested in working with them, and no more meetings with this particular person took place. At another meeting, where the researchers presented some of their findings, a member of the NHS England seemed unimpressed. He implied that some of the findings were irrelevant because they confirmed results already obtained through his own approach. Then he noted that another particular finding was irrelevant because it was different from what he had found.

Working with a large organisation can involve the navigation of complex human hierarchies where pre-existing and sometimes long-standing workplace rivalries and alliances are in existence and unlikely to be made transparent at the outset. Compatibility in terms of interaction style and personality might play a much larger role than expected in terms of whether an outside researcher will be accepted by members within the organisation. It should be borne in mind that there may be numerous elements of the ongoing relationship that researchers will have little control over.

During their presentations to NHS England, the researchers generally felt that their findings were taken seriously and welcomed, however. One of the presentations, involving a demonstration of a step-by-step corpus analysis of data, was recorded and placed on the NHS intranet system as training for others who wanted to follow the procedures. Team members who sat in on presentations were usually engaged, asking helpful questions or making useful observations at the end. However, it was seemingly difficult to evidence the impact that the CASS team's analysis had made on the organisation as a whole. For example, one of the research findings was that of all the different NHS staff members who received feedback from members of the public, receptionists received by far the worst forms of evaluation, often being described as rude or unhelpful, refusing to give appointments or asking invasive questions about patients' medical conditions. The analysis indicated that this was chiefly due to patients misunderstanding the roles of receptionists, who were implementing booking systems that they did not design, being sometimes required to ask questions about medical conditions in order to direct the patient to the most appropriate doctor. On the other hand, dentists often received extremely positive feedback from patients, but the researchers concluded that this was due to the fact that patients were often afraid of experiencing pain during a visit to the dentist, and when this did not happen, they were pleasantly surprised. Both the feedback regarding receptionists and dentists were governed by patient expectations which were not met. The team from CASS advised that rather than sending receptionists on social skills training courses, it would be sensible to engage in a public information campaign to educate people about receptionists' roles. It was also noted that a campaign to make people less afraid of dentists might *reduce* positive feedback about them, which raises an interesting dilemma.

These kinds of findings were received positively by the NHS England team, who reported how interesting they were, although it is not clear what they did with the information. It was not possible to ascertain the extent to which recommendations made by the CASS team would be implemented throughout the NHS, nor was it clear whether the methodological approaches that had been outlined to the team would be adopted to analyse subsequent sets of feedback. The NHS contact did provide a written statement outlining how useful the corpus approach and findings had been, which was used when reporting back to funders. The researchers also felt that they had made an impact on the NHS England team. However, the goal of showing that the NHS itself had changed as a result of our analysis was much more difficult to demonstrate, due to the unwieldly and nebulous nature of the large organisation and the length of time it can take for new recommendations to be implemented throughout a large organisation.

12.2.2 Disseminating Findings

In terms of wider dissemination, the findings were published as a monograph (Baker et al., 2019) and a journal article in the *British Medical Journal Open* (Brookes and Baker, 2017). The journal was targeted, as it was felt to be particularly likely to be read by medical practitioners, as opposed to academics. Additionally, the researchers used their university's press office to put out a press release about their findings on 2 May 2019.[1] This resulted in an article in *The Mail Online* (3 May 2019) which had an average daily readership of 2.18 million people between April 2019 and March 2020. Another article written by the team appeared in *The Conversation* (6 May 2019), which had a monthly readership of 10.7 million people in September 2019. The findings were also reported on several other websites, including Yahoo.com (6 May 2019), Practiceindex.co.uk

---

[1] www.lancaster.ac.uk/news/receptionists-take-the-everyday-flak-for-nhs-system-and-funding-issues.

(7 May 2019), *Metro* (7 May 2019; https://metro.co.uk), Dentistry.co.uk (9 May 2019), and *The Independent* (13 May 2019; www.independent.co.uk).

Writing a press release for a piece of corpus-based health research requires 'unlearning' some of the writing skills that have been accrued during an academic career. The press release that the researchers wrote was relatively short (760 words) and used non-technical language. Each sentence was written as separate paragraph. The researchers did not provide a summary of the entire project (which would have required answers to 12 research questions) but instead focussed on a single finding which was felt would be most interesting to the public. Galtung and Ruge's news values framework (1965) was considered in order to identify which of the findings would be likely to attract readers' attention. The pair of findings about people not liking receptionists but liking dentists was deemed to be a good possible story because it keyed into news values of negativity (people disliking receptionists), familiarity (most people have made an appointment to see a doctor), and unexpectedness (the reason why people thought receptionists were rude was not what we would expect). The researchers did not make any reference to corpus linguistics or technical terms like collocation, keywords, or concordances in the press release, as that would have required further explanation which would have detracted from the main point of the story. Instead, in the fourth paragraph the researchers wrote, 'The Lancaster University linguists used computer software to identify frequent or unusual patterns of language in the data but had to interpret the patterns themselves by reading hundreds of examples of feedback.'

Recommendations relating to a hypothetical public information campaign relating to receptionists were incorporated into the press release.

> 'Rather than suggesting that receptionists need retraining ... we instead noted that feedback is very much linked to expectations and constraints around different staff roles,' says Professor Paul Baker, who led the research.
>
> 'So jobs that involve saving your life or delivering a new life are seen as more impressive than the more support-based work carried out by nurses and receptionists – feedback has a role bias in other words.'
>
> The poorer evaluation of receptionists was strongly linked to people taking it personally when the receptionist could not give them an immediate appointment or was required to ask the patient questions to conduct triage.
>
> 'In other words they are often taking the flak for things that are not their fault but actually are indicative of patient frustration at bigger systemic issues – fewer appointments and longer waiting times are more likely to be the result of funding shortages that are beyond the receptionist's control,' added Professor Baker....
>
> 'Patients are then pleasantly surprised when the experience is not painful and so they leave excellent feedback as a result of their negative expectations not being met' explained Professor Baker. 'While this is good for dentists, it raises a dilemma if we simply measure NHS success in terms of patient ratings.

12.2 Working with an External Partner

'If the NHS embarked on awareness campaigns to counter fears about dentists, then more people would be likely to visit the dentist, although ultimately patients would be likely to end up being pleasantly surprised less, resulting in the amount of positive feedback around dentists perhaps going down over time.'

It could be argued that to an extent, the reporting of findings in the press release would have functioned as a public information campaign in its own right, as it would have been seen by potentially millions of people in the UK, from a range of different demographic groups. The aim in writing the press release was to encourage people to be less resentful (or abusive) towards receptionists and also be less afraid of visiting the dentist. However, while evidencing dissemination (how many people find out about a piece of research) is relatively easy, evidencing impact (the extent to which the research changes people's lives) can be more challenging. It would have taken a further study to investigate whether people's attitudes and behaviours towards receptionists and dentists had changed, and this was not something the researchers had funding to do, although for future projects it would be useful to consider how impact could be evidenced and to build this into funding proposals from the outset.

Finally, the researchers experienced an additional hurdle in the process of publishing findings when working with an external partner such as NHS England, which is somewhat different from working independently or with other academics. Publications needed to be signed off by the external partner. This process took longer than expected, particularly because with a large, complex organisation like the NHS, no single person was able to give permission to publish. Rather, the proposed publications were sent to multiple people at the NHS, who were all required to comment on them. Many of these people had other commitments and it was to their credit that they took the time to read the research drafts and provide their feedback and questions. For a later piece of research that the CASS team wanted to publish, the NHS used a staff member whose job was to ensure that the piece used language in a sensitive way, particularly relating to different identity groups. The paper to be published involved the analysis of language differences between men and women, and the NHS reader had quite specific requirements relating to how terms like *sex, gender, man, male, woman,* and *female* were used. This resulted in the terminology of the paper being changed accordingly, along with a delay, as the reader had numerous other documents to examine. It is therefore worth bearing in mind that publications resulting from collaboration with external partners may take longer to come to fruition than usual, particularly if the publications are to be submitted to journals and also reviewed by academics.

In summary, the collaboration with the NHS was one of the most rewarding pieces of research carried out within CASS, and it resulted in the research being among the most widely publicised, with articles in several national news outlets. This was also one of the first projects where members of CASS worked with an external partner. As noted, a key finding of the research was that the prior expectations of people who left feedback strongly impacted their responses, particularly in cases where these expectations did not meet reality. It is ironic, perhaps, that the researchers' own expectations of working with an external partner did not meet with reality, either. The researchers were treading uncharted territory during this project, and there was nobody who could advise on what their expectations should be and how to respond to the challenges that appeared. A lot of the time, the response involved improvisation or simply 'going with the flow' of the partner organisation. We hope that this section will alert readers to some of the possible ways that such a partnership might develop. However, we would not expect future research with external partners to work in the same way, and more than anything, we would advise analysts to expect the unexpected when working in similar contexts.

12.3 Disseminating the Findings of a Corpus-Based Project on Metaphors and Cancer

In this section we present some additional experiences of disseminating the findings of corpus-based research on health communication by referring to the Metaphor in End-of-Life Care' (MELC) project on metaphors and cancer, which has already been discussed in Chapters 5 and 9. In contrast with the example discussed in the previous section, the MELC project did not involve a collaboration with a single partner, but the funding for the project required interactions with stakeholders in cancer care and end-of-life care, as well as some evidence of what changes had resulted from these interactions.

As a reminder, the project was inspired by ongoing debates about the dominance and potential pitfalls, especially for patients, of metaphors whereby having cancer is presented as a fight or a battle with the disease – or, as the project team labelled them, Violence metaphors for cancer. The team combined manual analysis with the use of a range of corpus tools to study patterns in metaphor use in a 1.5-million-word corpus of interviews with and online writing by members of three different stakeholder groups in cancer care: patients, family carers, and healthcare professionals (Semino et al., 2018b).

As discussed in Chapter 9, the analysis provided evidence of the potentially harmful effects of Violence metaphors, particularly when a patient perceives themselves as responsible for 'losing the battle' when they have no prospect of recovery. However, a systematic analysis of occurrences of Violence metaphors in context revealed that, for some patients and depending on the

12.3 Disseminating the Findings of a Corpus-Based Project

circumstances, these metaphors can be empowering rather than disempowering. Indeed, the same observations about the importance of context and individual preferences and circumstances were found for Journey metaphors for cancer, which are sometimes perceived to be an alternative to Violence metaphors (e.g., 'my cancer journey'). The analysis of the MELC corpus revealed that Violence and Journey metaphors are the most frequent types of metaphors for all three groups of stakeholders in both genres represented in the corpus (Semino et al., 2018a). Eight additional main types of metaphors were also identified:

- Restraint: 'I feel like a prisoner with all the rules about don't eat this don't do that.'
- Animal: 'I am so sorry to hear that the beast is back.'
- Openness: 'From then on we were open we talked about it.'
- Sports and games: 'Caring for somebody with a terminal illness is more of a marathon rather than a sprint.'
- Religion and the supernatural: 'I just feel like a sitting duck waiting for the green eyed monster to come up and swallow me whole.'
- Obstacle: 'Add the dispensery [sic] pharmacist to the GP's receptionists and you've got the two big blockers to me getting what I need.'
- Wholeness: 'You realise you are only half a person.'
- Machine: 'I'm not really happy about being back on the treadmill of treatment.'

(Demjén and Semino, 2020: 195–6)

The project team was interdisciplinary. The Investigators included three linguists, a computer scientist, and a specialist in cancer and palliative care. In addition, the researchers regularly interacted with the Lancaster University Research Partner forum – a group of about a dozen people from northwest England with experience of cancer as patients or carers.

The MELC team aimed to disseminate the findings of the study to different academic audiences, including linguists and healthcare researchers, as well as to practitioners in healthcare and in cancer-related charities, in order to maximise the potential impact of the work on communication about cancer and the experiences of patients. To pursue this goal, they targeted journals from different disciplines as venues for publication and carried out a programme of engagement activities that included public lectures, training sessions for healthcare professionals and charity staff, blog posts, podcasts, and interactions with the media. This project therefore differed from the one described in the previous section, in that it was not commissioned by a specific stakeholder but rather aimed to reach a variety of different stakeholders, both proactively and, as the project became better known, reactively.

Broadly speaking, these goals were facilitated by the fact that the project involved large quantities of data and that the analysis was both quantitative and qualitative – in other words, by the adoption of corpus-based discourse analysis. This meant that the project could be taken seriously by audiences who favoured quantitative research on large datasets, as well as by audiences who favoured in-depth qualitative studies of authentic communication in context. In addition, the presence on the team of a highly respected healthcare researcher (Sheila Payne) led to initiatives that would have been difficult to achieve otherwise, because of the additional experience and credibility that this Co-investigator brought to the team. On the other hand, these goals were sometimes hampered by the fact that corpus linguistic methods were not known to many of the audiences targeted by the team, as well as by the lack of demographic information in the data from online forums. On many occasions, the team was asked whether there were any differences in metaphor use between men and women, older and younger people, people with different kinds or stages of cancer, and so on. When faced with these questions, the team could provide some general observations but no solid evidence of differences or lack of them, because of the anonymity afforded by the online forums from which data was drawn and the additional ethical guidelines that the project needed to follow in terms of anonymisation.

In the rest of this section we focus on three specific aspects of the project team's experiences in disseminating their findings beyond linguistics and beyond academia, and in trying to achieve concrete improvements in the support of patients and communication about cancer: writing for a healthcare journal, dealing with the media, and going beyond corpus data to create a metaphor-based resource for communication about cancer.

12.3.1 Writing for a Healthcare Journal

The project's findings were published in a monograph (Semino et al., 2018b), several linguistics journals (e.g., *International Journal of Corpus Linguistics* and *Applied Linguistics*; Demmen et al., 2015; Semino et al., 2018b), and one healthcare journal (*BMJ Supportive and Palliative Care*; Semino et al., 2017). This subsection is focused on the latter.

The original idea to publish some of the findings in *BMJ Supportive and Palliative Care* came from the healthcare researcher on the team, Sheila Payne. Payne suggested that the journal's readership would be interested in the quantitative and qualitative analyses of Violence and Journey metaphors in the data and particularly in the finding that the most crucial difference to be considered in communication about cancer is whether particular uses of metaphor are empowering or disempowering for patients in context, rather than what type of metaphors they are.

The biggest challenge at this point was to produce an article that followed the journal's guidelines, which were typical of healthcare and medical journals,

12.3 Disseminating the Findings of a Corpus-Based Project 195

particularly with regard to length. Linguistics journals typically have word count limits between 7,000 and 9,000 words for research articles. For *BMJ Supportive and Palliative Care*, however, the maximum length was 3,500 words. The lead author of the article and co-author of this book (Semino) struggled with producing a draft of the right length until Co-investigator Payne gave the following advice: 'Imagine a General Practitioner reading the article while eating a sandwich during their lunch break'. This advice helped Semino produce a draft of the appropriate length; it is also good advice generally, especially when writing for an audience outside one's discipline.

When it was submitted, the paper received largely favourable reviews. This was primarily because of the relevance of the findings to the journal's audience and because of the combination of quantitative and qualitative evidence from a large corpus that was mentioned earlier. This particular paper was in fact the most read in the journal for the first 12 months after publication, and at the time of this writing (April 2025) has more than 32,000 downloads.

Overall, corpus-based discourse analysis has considerable potential to cross disciplinary boundaries, as has been shown not just by this particular paper but also by articles published in a variety of journals by corpus linguists in our team at Lancaster and from many other institutions in the UK and across the world (e.g., Brookes and Baker, 2017; Jaworska, 2018). The effort involved in adapting to different academic conventions and different audiences is well worth it in terms of the additional reach and potential influence of the research findings.

12.3.2 Dealing with the Media

The MELC project attracted a considerable amount of media attention, with reports and interviews published in news outlets such as the *Daily Mail* in the UK and the *New York Times* in the US. This was a result of a combination of proactive initiatives on the part of the team and responses to media queries. For example, at an early point in the project, a press release was issued by the project's funders (the UK's Economic and Social Research Council) and Lancaster University. This led to several requests for interviews from national UK newspapers, as well as a couple of reproductions of the original press release in online outlets from different parts of the world. In other cases, media requests were received at times when communication about cancer, and specifically metaphors in communication about cancer, became topical, for example, when a celebrity or a politician used a particularly striking metaphor or explicitly rejected Violence metaphors for cancer.

Inevitably, journalists aimed to maximise the newsworthiness of the findings. However, in doing so, they sometimes misrepresented the research. Some of the misrepresentations were due to the attempt to simplify the message emerging from the research and confirm the audience's expectations about the negative consequences of Violence metaphors, in particular. For example, headlines would sometimes suggest that the project's main finding was that Violence metaphors should never be used, when in fact the analysis suggested that such metaphors can be both empowering and disempowering for patients:

> Mind your language: 'Battling' cancer metaphors can make terminally ill patients worse (*The Independent*, 3 November 2014)

> Cancer should not be called a 'battle' say language experts who fear metaphor makes people feel guilty if their condition gets worse (*The Daily Mail*, 4 November 2014)

The most extreme misrepresentation in this respect occurred in a book about metaphor and persuasion, where the author attributed to the project team the claim that people who used Violence metaphors had a poorer outlook than people who did not. This claim was such a serious and potentially dangerous misrepresentation of the project's findings that the team found a way to have it removed from the ebook version and subsequent print runs (Demjén and Semino, 2020).

A more specific kind of misrepresentation relates to the kind of data and findings that are typically involved in corpus linguistic projects. As corpus linguists, we typically use word counts or, even more precisely, token counts to report the size of corpora. This is not something that people outside our discipline are used to. For example, Demjén and Semino (2020) recall an occasion when a table reporting word counts for each of the sections of the MELC corpus initially caused some consternation (see Table 9.3). An audience of healthcare researchers interpreted figures over 80,000 in rows (within a table) corresponding to the interviews section of the corpus as reflecting the number of *interviews* that had been conducted, rather than the number of *words* in that section of the corpus. Something similar happened with the headline of an article in the *Mail Online*, which reported some project findings on the use of humorous metaphors in the data. The headline read:

> Laughter really is the best medicine for cancer patients: sufferers mock 'Mr C' to get through their illness and create a sense of community, reveals study of 1.5 million forum posts (6 December 2017)

In fact, the project team analysed a corpus of 1.5 million *words*, and while the number involved was reported accurately, the distinction between words and posts was lost on the journalists involved in producing the headline.

On a different occasion, the misrepresentation was more concerning. The Principal Investigator on the project (Semino) was interviewed by a *New York Times* journalist. The journalist was particularly interested in the finding that, in the corpus data, patients used Violence metaphors more frequently than healthcare professionals. When the article was published, the headline read:

> Fighting words are rarer among British doctors

Here the crucial point that the comparison was between British doctors and British patients was lost, and therefore the headline was interpreted as reflecting a comparison between British doctors and US doctors. This was, of course, inaccurate because the project did not involve a comparison between the UK and the US, never mind a finding concerning that particular difference. The mistake, we should add, was made by the sub-editor who created the headline. The writer of the piece was as distressed about the inaccuracy as the researchers were. Unfortunately, the headline was then picked up on Twitter, as it was then called, and that inaccurate finding was amplified. The project team therefore had to issue some clarification even though, in cases such as this, the clarification usually receives much less attention than the original misleading report. This whole incident actually then inspired the researchers to carry out the comparison that the headline assumed had already happened. That comparison did *not* in fact reveal a difference in the frequency of use of Violence metaphors between online writing produced by UK and US doctors (Potts and Semino, 2017).

12.3.3 Going beyond Corpus Data to Create a Communication Resource

The most enduring and successful outcome of the MELC project is a resource for communication about cancer called 'The Metaphor Menu for People Living with Cancer' (http://wp.lancs.ac.uk/melc/the-metaphor-menu/). This was not a planned output of the project. It was initially inspired by a question posed to the project team by a member of the previously mentioned Lancaster Research Partners Forum, along the lines of 'Are you going to produce something useful based on the research, such as a list of good and bad metaphors, so that people know what to do?'

When this question was asked in a meeting with the group, the project team replied by saying that this was not possible because the analysis had shown that the same metaphors work differently for different people, and that context makes a big difference in terms of whether a particular type of metaphor is empowering or disempowering. However, after more thought and discussion, the team came up with an idea that could meet the spirit if not the letter of the question.

The Metaphor Menu is a collection of 17 different metaphors for cancer, accompanied by images. They include some Violence and Journey metaphors, but also metaphors to do with nature, music, unwelcome visitors, and so on. The idea is not to prescribe which metaphors to use but to provide a wide range of possible metaphors as tools or resources for people to make sense of their experiences and to communicate about them, as well as inspiration to create their own metaphors. Indeed, the Metaphor Menu is precisely intended to suggest that different people may prefer different metaphors, and that the same metaphor will not appeal to everyone, as is the case with dishes on a restaurant menu.

The Metaphor Menu is recommended by Cancer Research UK and is being used in many different healthcare settings around the world. The process of selecting metaphors for inclusion, however, required considerable time and thought. The metaphors needed to be authentic (i.e., drawn from actual language use). Collectively, they needed to provide a wide variety of perspectives on cancer. They needed to be reasonably creative and striking. And, while they were not intended to sugar-coat the experience, they should also not be so negative as to potentially create distress. To achieve all these goals, even the variety of metaphors identified in the MELC corpus did not provide enough suitable candidates. Therefore, some of the metaphors in the Menu are from other sources, where the team had permission to include them. This flexibility was necessary to arrive at the best possible metaphor-based resource that could be created, even if it meant that the resource was not entirely based on corpus data.

Overall, the process of disseminating the findings of the MELC project was both challenging and rewarding, as with the NHS case study from the previous section. The MELC team has not initially expected both the challenges and opportunities that came their way, but the final outcomes were rewarding and worthwhile. Indeed, engagement with different stakeholders about the MELC findings is ongoing, and as we write this chapter, the Metaphor Menu is being extended as part of a new EU-funded project and versions of the Menu in other languages are being planned.

12.4 Conclusion

Looking back, the process of disseminating the findings of the two projects discussed in this chapter and throughout the book can be described as successful, in terms of publications within and outside linguistics, media reports, and even evidence of impact on, for example, practices in the NHS and communication about cancer. Indeed, these two specific projects were selected to be part of the 'impact' component of Lancaster University's linguistics submission to the 2021 'Research Excellence Framework' (REF, the national evaluation of research in the UK). That component was awarded the maximum score as part of the REF evaluation.

What we hope to have conveyed in this chapter, however, is what lies behind outcomes that can eventually be described as successful. As we have explained, dissemination beyond linguistics and beyond academia involved skills, situations, and activities that we, as corpus linguistics researchers, were not necessarily prepared for and did not always get right from the beginning, from coping with the turnover of people in a partner organisation to trying to write for healthcare audiences or the general public. We hope that by sharing the difficulties and compromises of our own experiences, we might prepare readers of this book for their own efforts, so that they can achieve their desired outcomes faster and more easily than we did. Overall, however, as we hope to have made clear, the hard work, setbacks, and compromises that we have described in this chapter were definitely worthwhile, and we all, as authors of this book, are proud of the reach and influence of CASS research on health communication over the years.

References

Baker, P., Brookes, G. and Evans, C. (2019). *The Language of Patient Feedback: A Corpus Linguistic Study of Online Health Communication*. Routledge.

Brookes, G. and Baker, P. (2017). What Does Patient Feedback Reveal about the NHS? A Mixed Methods Study of Comments Posted to the NHS Choices Online Service. *BMJ Open*, 7(4), e013821. https://doi.org/10.1136/bmjopen-2016-013821.

Demjén, Z. and Semino, E. (2020). Communicating Nuanced Results in Language Consultancy: The Case of Cancer and the Violence Metaphor. In L. Mullany (ed.), *Communicating in Professions and Organizations* (pp. 191–210). Palgrave.

Demmen, J., Semino, E., Demjén, Z., Koller, V., Payne, S., Hardie, H. and Rayson, P. (2015). A Computer-Assisted Study of Use of Violence Metaphors for Cancer and End of Life by Patients, Family Carers and Health Professionals. *International Journal of Corpus Linguistics*, 22(2), 205–31. https://doi.org/10.1075/ijcl.20.2.03dem.

Galtung, J. and Ruge, M. (1965). The Structure of Foreign News. The Presentation of the Congo, Cuba and Cyprus Crises in Four Norwegian Newspapers. *Journal of Peace Research*, 2(1), 64–91. https://doi.org/10.1177/002234336500200104.

Jaworska, S. (2018). Change but No Climate Change: Discourses of Climate Change in Corporate Social Responsibility Reporting in the Oil Industry. *International Journal of Business Communication*, 55(2), 194–219. https://doi.org/10.1177/2329488417753951.

McIntyre, D. and Price, H. (eds.) (2018). *Applying Linguistics: Language and the Impact Agenda*. Routledge.

(eds.) (2023). *Public Linguistics: Communicating Language Research beyond Academia*. Routledge.

Mullany, L. (ed.) (2020). *Professional Communication: Consultancy, Advocacy, Activism*. Palgrave.

Potts, A. and Semino, E. (2017). Healthcare Professionals' Online Use of Violence Metaphors for Care at the End of Life in the US: A Corpus-Based Comparison with the UK. *Corpora*, 12(1), 55–84. https://doi.org/10.3366/cor.2017.0109.

Semino, E., Demjén, Z. and Demmen, J. (2018a). An Integrated Approach to Metaphor and Framing in Cognition, Discourse and Practice, with an Application to Metaphors for Cancer. *Applied Linguistics*, 39(5), 625–45. https://doi.org/10.1093/applin/amw028.

Semino, E., Demjén, Z., Demmen, J., Koller, V., Payne, S., Hardie, H. and Rayson, P. (2017). The Online Use of 'Violence' and 'Journey' Metaphors by Cancer Patients, as Compared with Health Professionals: A Mixed Methods Study. *BMJ Supportive and Palliative Care*, 7(1), 60–6. https://doi.org/10.1136/bmjspcare-2014-000785.

Semino, E., Demjén, Z., Hardie, A., Rayson, P. and Payne, S. (2018b). *Metaphor, Cancer and the End of Life: A Corpus-Based Study*. Routledge.

13 Conclusions

13.1 Introduction

In this final chapter of the book, we present a synthesis of the previous chapters. We first consider the question: what are the key insights into health communication that our different projects have given us? We then move on to consider the lessons we learned about carrying out corpus-based research on health communication, offering practical advice and tips relating to research questions, datasets, analytical approaches, and going beyond academia. This is followed by a section which critically considers the limitations of the corpus-based approach. And, finally, we consider future directions for corpus-assisted healthcare research, asking what has changed since we completed the projects described in this book and what avenues of research we believe are potentially interesting to investigate next.

13.2 What Have We Learnt about Health Communication That We Did Not Know Before?

In this section, rather than reiterating some of the main findings from the parts of individual studies described in earlier chapters, we instead want to focus on some of our 'bigger picture' findings, which tend to stretch across and connect with multiple projects.

First, health communication is not restricted to health practitioners or even communication between health practitioners and patients. In particular, people who experience health conditions are not passive – they co-construct understandings around their conditions on their own terms, without their medical practitioners. The data we examined was incredibly *human*. We found human nature displayed in comedic or cute ways when finding metaphors to frame health conditions – from the long-running humorous reframing of cancer patients as members of an army to the creation of a cartoon-like 'Mr Anxiety'. We found that human nature could sometimes be articulated through fear or prejudice – from concerns that a vaccination might kill you to the characterisation of syphilis as a 'French' disease. And there were even aspects of human nature that manifested as entitled or petty – from a patient's complaint that they expected better treatment because their family had lived in the same area for hundreds of years through to news articles gloating about murderers putting on weight in prison. For some of us, prior to working with corpora of health data, we had expected that we would be analysing a very dry, scientific form of discourse. This was rarely the case. Sometimes the texts we read could be extremely funny, frustrating, or moving. The data was thus much more engaging than expected, although that could also bring challenges with it, especially when the material was potentially distressing and we were aiming for as much objectivity as possible in our approach to it.

Collectively, the corpora collected for our projects show how health communication extends across a much wider range of linguistic 'events' than, say, an appointment with a General Practitioner. People gain understandings about health from a wide variety of sources: friends and family, online forums, governments, scientific researchers and the media, and these sources interact with one another – nobody can be said to be truly impartial or beyond influence from the discourses of others. Although health conditions are real and exist beyond discourse (as cancer and COVID-19 can kill people), the ways that we understand and react to them are dependent on discourse, and language plays a major role in conveying, challenging, and upholding these different understandings. Language is where we co-construct beliefs about what counts as a health condition and what counts as healthy. And there is a lot more variation than we had expected to find – for example, when we observed that Violence metaphors for cancer seem to be empowering for some patients. Fortunately, a corpus-based approach is well-suited to explore and identify a lot of this variation. With millions of words of naturally occurring data, we were able to confidently make generalisations about trends in language use, while also spotting the less frequent patterns which may have been missing from smaller datasets.

Similarly, the ways that we use language to communicate about health are varied – in some of our projects we took a prospective view, allowing different forms of language to emerge during our analyses. We had not expected there to be so many metaphors across different projects, but there was also abundant use of transitivity, evaluation, legitimation, narrative, humour, punning, emojis, alliteration, and anthropomorphisation. The authors of this book all have backgrounds in linguistics, which proved to be helpful in identifying the wide range of phenomena encountered throughout the different corpora, but even we were surprised by the extent of linguistic variation across each project. With each new corpus, we had to set aside what we had done and start again, with fresh eyes.

One aspect of our research that we had not expected to play such an important role was identity. A lot the variation that we found can be accounted

13.3 Advice for Corpus Researchers in Health Communication 203

for through identity variables – it predicted differences in language use in patient feedback and in the ways that people on online forums framed their health conditions. It also played a key role in the ways that journalists wrote about health – obesity is *very* gendered in the news. We all hold multiple identities, which can shift in and out of focus in different contexts, like kaleidoscope patterns. Some identity characteristics can be easier to identify and compare than others, though; the challenge for analysts is to consider which ones are most relevant and which are missing but ought to be interrogated. We also need to consider which identities interact together (sex *and* age helped explain variation in patient feedback relating to cancer, for example). Another key factor in terms of variation is time, and our analyses have shown how the consideration of time can go beyond merely dividing a corpus up into years based on date of publication of texts but can also involve annual patterns, the age of the contributor, or the length of time they have spent in a particular discourse community.

Health communication research can perhaps be characterised as action-oriented, in that it aims to improve understandings of language use around health in order to foster better health outcomes for people. Many researchers in this field (particularly the subfield of corpus-based health research) tend to take a descriptive rather than an evaluative view. Often, we do not know what we are going to find in a corpus, and so we generally do not set out to 'prove a point' or be critical of people's language use. So, in our analyses of metaphors around cancer, we created a metaphor menu as opposed to suggesting that some metaphors were bad, while in our analyses of an anxiety forum, we were cautious about suggesting that some framings of anxiety were harmful. On the other hand, in some of our projects, we have tried to offer more direct advice – such as making suggestions to improve the descriptors used in the pain questionnaire, consider how the NHS could use information campaigns to change patient expectations, or determine how journalists could write about people with obesity or dementia in ways that are less stigmatising. The answer to the question of what to do with a finding also varied tremendously across our projects. While Chapter 2 outlines the ways we created research questions under different conditions, a point to bear in mind is that all of these projects had a similar overall goal – how to do the most good. This was not a question we explicitly considered when we were focussed on each project, but in hindsight, we realise it is the most important one.

13.3 What Advice Would We Pass on to Other Corpus Researchers Working in Health Communication?

When you read an account of a research project in an academic journal, book, or newspaper report, it has usually been tidied up – with false starts, backtracks, dead ends, and loose endings all made magically invisible, as if they never happened. In other words, this is often a simplified version of what actually happened. Projects are rarely like that, though. They can be messy and even go horribly wrong in both foreseen and unexpected ways. In some of the worst cases, they can fail to produce anything of value. The projects we described in this book *were* successful, although they did not always go as planned. So, with the accumulated knowledge of all these projects, what tips would we give to other corpus researchers in health communication? What do we wish we had known from the start?

First, corpus research in health communication is often best achieved through teamwork. The approach requires quite a wide-ranging skill set, and it is unlikely that a single person will be able to tick every box on the list. Computational knowledge is useful for building, cleaning, and annotating corpora, then mounting it on analysis software. Statistical skills are required to make sense of what the tests are doing, which ones should be used, and what the settings should be. Linguistic skills are needed in order to identify and interpret the features in a corpus. Depending on the corpus under examination, we may also need a specialist historian or someone with detailed knowledge about a particular social or political context. And it is also very important to involve someone with knowledge about the particular health condition or healthcare setting. All of the corpus-based projects we describe in this book involved more than one person, and frequently, they involved someone who was *not* a corpus linguist. It perhaps seems counter-intuitive to say that a corpus project should actively seek to recruit someone who is not knowledgeable about corpus linguistics, but for health-related communication, there are advantages to be gained. The non–corpus linguist can provide a better sense of what matters in the health-based context under examination. They can give the research a clearer and more relevant focus, and help interpret and explain results. As we saw in Chapter 2, they can also push corpus linguists out of their analytical comfort zone, ensuring that they are not stuck doing repetitive 'handle-turning' forms of research. Thus, we would advise viewing this kind of research as a continuing dialogue between multiple participants with different areas of expertise. However, as Chapter 12 showed, relationships between those working in academia and those connected to health organisations do not always go as planned. Therefore, the dialogue should also involve a focus on scheduling and dividing tasks, allowing the different parties to compare their organisational structures in order to set expectations and boundaries. This might save time and avoid disappointment at a later date.

In terms of creating a corpus, it is important to consider what any initial research questions are and not to spend so long creating the perfect corpus that there is a suboptimal amount of time required to analyse it – even if this means collecting less data or tolerating a certain level of messiness in the corpus itself,

13.3 Advice for Corpus Researchers in Health Communication 205

as with the OCR errors in the VicVaDis corpus. Unless you are certain that a hand-annotated corpus is required, this is probably not something to embark on at the outset; you can also add in those annotations later if they become essential. Some form of automatic tagging can be a more pragmatic option initially, although we would advise analysts to be mistrustful of the accuracy of automatic tags; for example, when working with a grammatical tagged version of the news corpus on obesity, we found numerous cases of the word *fat* tagged as an adjective when it should have been a noun. Such cases had to be weeded out by hand, and if we had just taken the cases at face value, we would have achieved very different (and much less accurate) results. Expect that there will be both anticipated and unanticipated tagging errors and keep an eye out for them, making adjustments to your calculations if and when needed.

A pilot analysis can be useful in terms of helping spot potential problems with a corpus. Even when we worked with corpora that had not been tagged, we discovered numerous instances of duplicated files or unwanted boilerplates (such as repeated menu headings from websites or copyright information) which skewed frequencies and gave us keywords and collocates that were less accurate or useful than they should have been. Be prepared *not* to trust your text, in other words, and to view the initial analyses more as troubleshooting exercises, aimed at weeding out these kinds of problems with data collection.

Some forms of corpora bring with them their own challenges. Spoken corpora are especially time-consuming to collect and transcribe, in addition to posing some of the most complex ethical challenges involving anonymisation and consent. When working with most health-based topics, it is important to take ethics into account (with exceptions such as texts widely intended for public consumption like newspaper articles), and this may mean that there are some forms of data that simply can't be collected or that we can't have full knowledge of. For example, with the forum posts on pain and anxiety, some posters had not consented to their data being used for research, so their posts had been removed in advance of us receiving the data. When working with data of an interactive nature, this reduces the kinds of analysis we can confidently carry out, and sometimes we have to accept that what we have is not ideal – although it can still tell us other things. Ethics aside, one concerning aspect that we noted while we worked on these projects is that some forms of data are becoming more difficult to obtain; X (formerly Twitter) has placed restrictions on how its social media posts can be collected, while the LexisNexis online news aggregator has undergone several changes to its database in recent years. At one point, the site required users to manually tick a check box for each article they wanted to collect. More recently, the database has limited the number of articles that can be collected in one day to 1,000. Owners of online data are understandably concerned about mass scraping of their data, which has sometimes been used without permission in large language models for AI chatbots. The larger point we want to make is that data collection protocols can change rapidly. Don't assume, from reading about one of the studies in this book, that your experience of collecting data will be the same.

For our projects involving corpora of speech, such as Emergency Departments conversations or interviews relating to voice-hearing, we had to rely solely on human transcribers – although more recently new technologies have helped improve transcription, both in terms of speed and cost. For example, Sonix[1] is an online audio and video transcription software which we have since used in other corpus projects. The tool does not provide 100 per cent accuracy, but it greatly reduces the amount of work that human transcribers need to do. Mobile phone technology has become much more impressive over the past decade – point a phone at a page of printed text and its camera can likely scan and create an electronic version of it. Even handwritten pages can be converted in this way, although they tend to be less accurately rendered. When reading about how others created corpora, don't assume that the technology has stood still and you should replicate older methods of data collection. The same point applies to corpus analysis tools; during the period in which we worked on these projects, newer versions of existing tools were launched, enabling a wider range of forms of analysis. While it is important, then, to refer to existing literature, this is a field which is moving quickly – a warning that by the time any piece of corpus research has been published, it is already out of date.

Readers of this book will have noticed that we did not rely on a single corpus tool for all our projects, but we used a variety of them: Sketch Engine, AntConc, CQPweb, WordSmith, and Wmatrix. In some cases, choice of software was governed by our existing familiarity with certain tools; in others, it was influenced by the different affordances that tools allow. Sometimes multiple tools needed to be used with the same corpus, although it should be borne in mind that slightly different results can be obtained. For example, different tool creators might have their own views on how to define a 'token' (some may advocate splitting hyphenated words into two tokens, some may not), and this can impact on frequency counts. In addition, some tools may have different means of calculating collocation or keyness. Aim for consistency, if possible, and be clear about which tool was used for each procedure.

The different chapters across this book have also indicated that there is no single approach or pathway to carrying out analysis. Instead, we are given a bunch of analytical techniques and can choose to apply some or all of them in different orders, using different cut-off points or tests for statistical significance. The lack of a single route can be challenging but also liberating – enabling

---

[1] https://sonix.ai/.

13.3 Advice for Corpus Researchers in Health Communication

a more experimental, ludic approach to analysing a corpus. It can be helpful, at least at first, to try to take into account the goals of the project as well as the nature of the corpus. Sometimes we might want to focus on a single word or phrase in the corpus which is considered to be important (such as the word *anxiety* or *pain*). In other cases, we may want to look at the corpus as a whole. Sometimes we may decide in advance which kinds of linguistic features we want to examine – such as metaphors – while in other cases we might want to allow salient or frequent linguistic features to emerge. There are advantages and limitations to both approaches, and a certain amount of reflective modesty is advised when outlining findings and implications. Of course, there is no reason why a combination of approaches cannot be taken, and sometimes shifting between a mixture of targeted and prospective techniques can work well.

Another piece of advice we would give is to be prepared to change course, to allow the corpus analysis to reveal new and unexpected avenues. Be on the lookout for answers to questions that you did not think of but are actually more interesting than the ones you originally asked. For example, in the study on venereal disease discussed in Chapter 8, analysis of collocates revealed so many place names that this shifted the nature of the research. And in the study on patient feedback from Chapter 6, the analysts gradually realised that the nature of the data involved a lot of legitimation alongside the evaluation – legitimation that lent itself to questions that neither the corpus linguists nor the NHS team had originally thought of.

Another piece of advice we can't stress enough is to avoid making assumptions about decontextualised language use. You are likely to be looking at a lot of lists of words and phrases with numbers alongside them. We might be tempted to guess at what these words mean or imply for our data, but experience has shown us again and again that we can often be completely wrong. This is a case where we need to trust the *context* – reading concordance lines, sometimes expanded concordance lines, in order to truly get a sense of how a linguistic item is being used. It is worth trying to achieve a balance between covering lots of linguistic items while also getting a reasonably accurate account of them. If a word occurs 20,000 times in your corpus, we would advise that it is not a good use of your time (and sanity) to look through all 20,000 lines. In many cases, examining a random selection of 100 lines is likely to identify the main trends. If this provides inconclusive results, the selection can be expanded. A thousand lines is likely to give a good selection of rarer cases (although not all the rare cases).

Corpus research is especially well-suited to impact the world outside of academia. The sheer size of our datasets enables our findings to be taken seriously, while our combination of quantitative and qualitative approaches means that we often have opportunities to make unexpected insights into language use. The challenge, then, is in conveying our findings to those outside academia – particularly as this is an area where we may not have as much experience or training. Be mindful that an academic style is unlikely to be appropriate for most forms of impact. In this book we have written about unlearning academic writing skills and thinking about specific audiences (in some cases very specific – say a General Practitioner reading while eating a sandwich for lunch). Rather than crossing one's fingers and hoping that our attempts to communicate outside our domain will work, it is worth spending some time reading existing news articles and press releases that discuss health-related or corpus-based academic research, while critically engaging with them to get a sense of what works. Non-academic members of a research team can be especially valuable in helping frame these kinds of dissemination texts, while also ensuring that the style is appropriate. Short, unambiguous, surprising messages tend to work well, so be sure to get advice if this style of writing is not your forte and consider some media training if you are going to be giving interviews as well. Also, heed a warning from Chapter 12: it is worth considering the ways that your message might get mangled. If possible, ask a journalist to send a copy of their news story back to you, prior to publication (and raise a red flag if they are reluctant to do so).

13.4 What Are the Limitations of the Corpus-Based Approach?

No approach can do everything well, and we hope that this book has given readers a sense of where the corpus approach can shine and where it can only take us so far.

One limitation relates to the kinds of data that are available to us in large enough amounts for a corpus approach to be considered. While even a small data set can be referred to as a corpus, a few thousand words is likely to be short enough for a qualitative close reading to be carried out on it, and unless the corpus contains a lot of lexical repetition, frequencies are unlikely to be high enough for much of interest to emerge through techniques like keywords or collocation.

Some texts are easier to collect than others, which can push analysis into certain directions and away from others. Written data is usually easier to source than spoken data. Recent data is easier than historic data (as a general rule, the further back in time you go, the harder it is to build a corpus). Spoken historical data can be extremely difficult to find. Online data can be an easier option, then, although even here there can be potential access difficulties, and the presence of bots can sometimes make us question the veracity of such data. Note that large amounts of text can bring their own problems. Some analysis tools will crash or work very slowly when working with millions or billions of words of data. And the more text we have, the harder it is to fully understand, risking errors of interpretation.

13.4 What Are the Limitations of the Corpus-Based Approach?

The bedrock of the corpus approach is frequency, and that can reveal a great many insights, although not all. Some things are more difficult to identify and count than others; hence there can be a risk that we limit our analyses to simple word frequencies, as opposed to, say, more complex and variable phenomena like metaphor or joking.

Two corpora may have similar relative frequencies of a word, but in each corpus that word might be used very differently – something which we may miss if we only carry out a keywords analysis. And techniques like keywords prompt us to consider frequency differences as being important; they often are, but it might be the case that the *similarities* between two corpora are also relevant. Frequency can also make us focus on presence – we may spend so long counting what is in a corpus that we don't notice what isn't there. So think about the *absence* of linguistic features as well as presence. What could be there, or should be there, but isn't? It is thus worth reflecting on how the analytical methods you employ might be limiting you or steering you in certain directions. Comparing frequencies across multiple corpora might help identify the complete absence of a feature in one of them, but what if the feature occurs in none of the corpora?

We advise researchers to consider whether a corpus approach is actually going to enable you to answer your research questions effectively. In some of the studies we outlined in this book, we concluded that using tools like collocation and keywords alone would not get us far, so we switched to a more qualitative, manual analysis (e.g., the annotation of discourse functions in the anxiety forum corpus, as well as the identification of metaphor in the MELC corpus). While such approaches can be time-consuming, they don't necessarily need to involve the entire corpus – sometimes a downsampled set will provide enough evidence for us to be able to spot trends or carry out comparisons of the most frequent features, even if we can't say that the analysis will be exhaustive.

The techniques of corpus linguistics are descriptive. They can tell us what is happening with language, but they can't tell us what this means, or why it is happening, or whether this should be happening. In contexts like health communication, the corpus approach needs supplementing with consideration of relevant forms of context so we can interpret, explain, and critique the findings. So, for example, the analysis of the newspaper corpus of articles about obesity revealed the ways that journalists write negatively about people with obesity, using shaming and ridiculing language. However, the corpus analysis alone can't tell us why journalists did that. We would need to think more about the context of news reporting in the country and time period under study, along with taking into account aspects like government policy, press regulation, readership demographics, and vested economic concerns. In interpreting and evaluating our findings, we might want to consult with stakeholder groups who are likely to be able to offer real-world insights based on lived experience.

13.5 Final Thoughts: What about the Future?

The projects described in this book ran between the years 2012 and 2023, with the most recent corpus texts being in data from Mumsnet, which includes contributions posted up to the end of 2022. What changes have taken place since that period that are relevant for health communication? In the UK there have been unprecedented decreases in satisfaction with the NHS – from an average 53 per cent satisfaction in 2020 to 24 per cent in 2023.[2] Our two patient feedback studies covered earlier time periods, where we found a mostly positive picture. The change indicates how time-limited such research can be, as well as the need to continue analysing feedback data in order to respond to contexts that are in constant flux.

Linked to changes in patient satisfaction, the political context has also changed. For our study on press language around obesity, we collected news articles published between 2008 and 2017. The majority of the articles in that corpus, then, had been written under a Conservative-led government in the UK. Perhaps unsurprisingly, we found that news framings about obesity tended to be largely congruent with the dominant political ideologies of the time, for example, by stressing personal contexts while reducing the role of larger social structures. Consequently, there had been a move away from discussing obesity in terms of issues like inequality and poverty, despite the fact that such phenomena had increased over the period under study. In 2024, a Labour government came to power; shifts in terms of the ideologies and policies of those who run a country tend to impact on health policy, and it will be interesting to see how a new set of leaders will influence language use relating to health, not just in the press but in a wide range of communicational contexts.

There have also been changes in terms of a biomedical perspective. Sticking with obesity – in 2022, a review of anti-obesity treatments concluded that semaglutide (an antidiabetic medication) was more promising than previous anti-obesity drugs, and in 2023, a brand of the drug called Wegovy was approved for use by the NHS for weight loss. Demand for such drugs appears to be rising, popularised by celebrity endorsements – particularly in the US. *The New York Times* published an opinion piece on 23 October 2023 which claimed 'these drugs are blockbusters because they promise to solve a medical problem that is also a cultural problem – how to cure the moral crisis of fat

---

[2] https://natcen.ac.uk/publications/public-attitudes-nhs-and-social-care#:~:text=In%202023%2C %20fewer%20than%201,public%20satisfaction%20with%20the%20NHS.

bodies that refuse to get and stay thin'.[3] It isn't difficult to see how scientific advances can completely change the discourses around health conditions. These examples show how research which looks at health communication in contemporary contexts needs to be ongoing in order to keep up with relevant developments in a quickly changing world. As noted earlier, frustratingly, by the time that a corpus has been created and analysed, and the research published, it can already feel slightly out of date. This is less the case for research which considers historical contexts, like the studies on venereal disease and vaccine hesitancy discussed in Chapter 8, and it is interesting to see how centuries-old texts can still shed light on the present day. Consequently, corpus studies using recent data, while situating the findings within that context, should also articulate more solid and lasting findings and implications from their projects.

Artificial intelligence and systems like ChatGPT appear, on face value, to be able to answer any question or analyse any text which is presented to them. These systems were not available when we carried out our corpus research, which involved a lot of human-led decision-making, analysis, and interpretation. Since then, ChatGPT has been incorporated into AntConc, and some of us have experimented with the potential for AI tools to aid in corpus analysis (see Curry et al., 2024), finding a mixed picture (i.e., not one in which we believe AI could replace human researchers, at least not at this point in time). ChatGPT did a reasonable job of putting keywords into thematic categories but had difficulty in interpreting concordance lines where knowledge of context was required. Broadly, it could produce a piece of corpus research which might achieve a low pass mark if submitted as an undergraduate essay but would not be publishable.

On the whole, though, computational advances present opportunities for corpus researchers. Often the texts that are taken to be compiled into a corpus are a mixture of writing and images, with the latter elements usually stripped out (such was the case for the obesity news corpus). However, AI tools are becoming adept at tagging images with labels, based on millions of cases of existing pre-tagged data. We have experimented with one tool (Vertex AI, formerly called Google Cloud Vision), working with a small corpus of news articles about obesity (Baker and Collins, 2023). Incorporating image tags into the corpus allows the analysis to be truly multimodal. For example, we were able to consider which newspapers tended to use which types of images and the extent to which particular words appeared in articles that contained certain images. Our analysis helped us show how stories that sympathetically focussed on people's struggles with obesity tended to show them in formalwear at public events, whereas those which focussed on body positivity were more likely to

---

[3] www.nytimes.com/2023/10/09/opinion/ozempic-obesity-fat-diabetes.html.

have pictures of women in revealing clothing. There is a great deal of potential, then, for corpus analyses to consider the relationship between words and image.

It is challenging to try to identify future topics, even when extrapolating from current trends. For example, improved healthcare across the globe is helping to increase lifespan, which is likely to have implications for the kinds of health care that will be needed and talked about. In recent years, there have been greater numbers of people reporting mental health problems over time, as well as more people diagnosed with forms of neurodiversity. Both indicate future avenues of health communication research to be explored. Additionally, rising average global temperatures due to humanity's burning of fossil fuels are likely to result in increases in a range of different health conditions, such as Lyme disease, West Nile virus, cardiovascular disease, allergies, and asthma, in addition to impacts on mental health. Another pandemic is possible in the not-too-distant future, while advances in immunotherapy for cancer are beginning to involve personalised 'vaccines' that train the immune system to recognise and kill the patient's cancer cells. Increased automatisation of healthcare through AI and robotics is also likely to suggest new directions for analysis. For example, an offshoot of our corpus analysis of the anxiety forum involved us collaborating with the charity Anxiety UK in order to analyse human interactions with a chatbot on its website; corpus analysis helped us discuss with the charity how the chatbot's responses could be improved (Collins et al., 2024).

Finally, the research outlined in this book was carried out at a British university with funding from UK funders and mainly had a British focus, with some exceptions (the Emergency Departments corpus contained Australian data, while the health and pain forums contained significant amounts of posts written by American authors). On the whole, however, we have focussed on the UK and the English language – taking advantage of our familiarity with this context, which helped in terms of providing interpretations and explanations of our findings. We want to make it clear, though, that the techniques described in this book can be used with all languages, and we would hope to encourage future researchers to carry out corpus-based analyses of health communication in an ever-broadening range of geopolitical and historical contexts. There is also much to be gained from research which takes comparable datasets from different countries and time periods, identifying differences and similarities and basing interpretations on different social, political, and economic contexts and how they intersect with understandings of health. It should not be assumed that such projects will be straightforward in terms of locating and gaining access to data. The political systems in some countries may make it harder to gain access to certain kinds of health-related texts. Similarly, in some countries it can be difficult to publish anything which might be interpreted as being critical of the government, with resulting

13.5 Final Thoughts: What about the Future?

implications for objectivity. The Global Expression Report (2023) found that only 13 per cent of the world's population live in 'open' countries, while 34 per cent of people live in countries where freedom of expression is in crisis. There needs to be more thought and effort to enable health communication research to represent the health experiences and concerns of the whole world.

In closing, we hope that this collection has helped provide a sense of the scope and techniques associated with a corpus-based approach to health communication. We also hope that we have conveyed the value and importance of this approach. Our aim in writing this book has been to encourage and inspire others to work in this field – all the studies that we describe here were both challenging and rewarding, and we feel that we have learnt a lot from our experiences and grown as researchers. Our team started from a relative position of ignorance, with a steep learning curve. Our goal is to hopefully make that learning curve a little less daunting for others.

References

Baker, P. and Collins, L. (2023). Creating and Analysing a Multimodal Corpus of News Texts with Google Cloud Vision's Automatic Image Tagger. *Applied Corpus Linguistics*, 3(1), 100043. https://doi.org/10.1016/j.acorp.2023.100043.

Collins, L., Nicholson, N., Lidbetter, N., Smithson, D. and Baker, P. (2024). Implementation of Anxiety UK's Ask Anxia® Chatbot Service: Lessons Learned. *JMIR Human Factors*, 11, e53897. https://doi.org/10.2196/53897.

Curry, N., Baker, P. and Brookes, G. (2024). Generative AI for Corpus Approaches to Discourse Studies: A Critical Evaluation of ChatGPT. *Applied Corpus Linguistics*, 4(1), 10082. https://doi.org/10.1016/j.acorp.2023.100082.

Global Express Report. (2023). *Article 19*. www.article19.org/resources/the-global-ex pression-report-2023/?gad_source=1&gclid=Cj0KCQjw0ruyBhDuARIsANSZ3 wobAv2bd1ZAjE41VoGcRox-BWpiXfmET7CO1NY6uoJ_bLsOAVH4tRsaAn2 vEALw_wcB.

Index

advice, 80, 114, 115
advice-giving, 82
age, 45, 86, 90, 93, 112, 114, 180, 182
agency, 55, 70, 128, 138, 145, 150, 153, 161, 162, 165, 177
annotation, 41, 69, 85, 88, 97, 205
anonymity, 41, 55, 56, 59, 194
AntConc, 120, 122, 211
anthropomorphism, 139, 140
anxiety disorders, 74, 81, 112, 114, 116, 134, 143
artificial intelligence (AI), 211
  chatbot, 208, 212
  ChatGPT, 155, 211

Biber, D., 35, 77, 79
blame, 29, 124, 129
boilerplate, 38, 205

cancer, 69, 73, 105, 125, 143, 146, 148, 192
  cancer care, 87, 150
  cervical cancer, 120
charity, 58, 71, 212
co-design, 62, 63, 64
coefficient of variation, 102
collocation, 5, 24, 28, 114, 120, 127, 130, 135, 136, 138, 156, 157, 164
compulsory vaccination, 6, 47, 118, 120, 122, 178
concordance, 72, 89, 104, 107, 127, 146, 156, 159, 207, 211
conflict, 171
consent, 41, 57, 58, 61, 64, 205
conversation analysis, 43, 69, 94
corpus design, 34, 37
corpus query, 43, 45, 156, 157, 164, 173
corpus software, 3, 116, 126, 206
corpus-assisted discourse analysis, 17, 28, 30
COVID-19, 47, 122, 124, 125, 130, 177
CQPweb, 38, 41, 45, 89, 126, 156, 157
crime, 159

demographic metadata, 60, 86, 88, 91, 94, 98
diagnosis, 20, 23, 61
diet, 18, 110
discourse prosody, 114, 136, 141
discourse unit, 9, 77, 79
dissemination, 41, 59, 186, 189, 191, 192, 208

Early English Books Online (EEBO), 126
Emergency Departments (EDs), 40
exercise, 112, 159
eXtensible Markup Language (XML), 41, 44

food, 107, 156
framing, 109, 129
frequency, 24, 36, 38, 43, 45, 102, 103, 164, 206, 209
  frequency list, 4, 155
funding, 60, 186, 191

genre, 24, 49, 122, 128
geographical information systems, 127
government, 109, 111, 178, 210
grammatical categories, 136, 156
guidelines, 61, 64, 138, 194

Halliday, M., 153, 162, 164
health communication, 2, 9, 33, 39, 87, 170, 201, 204
health system, 74, 90
healthcare professionals, 2, 56, 147
  dental practice, 180, 182, 189, 191
  receptionist, 188, 190
HealthUnlocked, 58, 59
historical data, 34, 36, 46, 50, 56, 118
humour, 70, 71, 72, 74, 148

information campaign, 189, 190
Institute for Communication in Health Care (ICH), 40, 41
Islam, 18, 154

214

Index

justice, 55, 65

keyness, 6, 71, 101, 102, 113, 155, 209
  key semantic domains, 71
keywords, 6, 88, 94, 107, 110, 122, 211
  remainder method, 107, 110, 113, 155

legitimation, 29, 96, 169, 170, 176, 178, 179, 182
lexis, 4, 18, 21, 103, 106, 119, 135, 142
LexisNexis, 35, 36, 38, 154
lifestyle, 108, 121
lived experience, 62, 68, 143, 210

McGill Pain Questionnaire (MPQ), 20, 23, 24, 25
metadata, 38, 41, 46, 75, 86, 93, 128
metaphor, 21, 69, 73, 74, 121, 138, 158, 195
  army metaphor, 71, 73, 143
  battle metaphor, 69, 73, 74, 140, 142, 143, 144, 148, 149, 192, 196
  Journey metaphor, 70, 105, 116, 140, 144, 145, 146, 193
  metaphor identification, 145, 146
  Violence metaphor, 70, 145, 146, 148, 192
Metaphor in End-of-Life Care (MELC), 69, 144, 148, 192, 195, 197
Mumsnet, 171, 173

narrative, 159, 177
nationality, 128
news, 17, 35, 36, 102, 154, 195, 209, 210, 211
  annual news cycle, 18, 106, 110
  broadsheet, 19
  Daily Mail, 36, 189, 196
  journalism, 109, 190, 195, 196, 203, 209
  tabloids, 19, 37, 158
nomination, 155

obesity, 18, 19, 108, 112, 154, 157, 210
online support group, 56, 58, 59, 60, 68, 71, 74, 77, 112, 134, 171, 205
optical character recognition (OCR), 50
Oxford English Corpus (OEC), 23

pain, 20, 59, 96, 182
patient feedback, 26, 87, 102, 183
personification, 71, 138, 149, 161
policy, 109, 111, 144
pox, 47, 119, 127
process types, 162, 165
psychosis, 160, 165
  auditory verbal hallucinations, 160

qualitative analysis, 2, 5, 40, 159, 183

representativeness, 35, 37, 50, 98
risk, 56, 119, 121

secondary analysis, 39, 40
semantic domains, 71, 106, 145
sex and gender, 86, 88, 94, 96, 158, 182, 191
  female, 88, 91, 95
  male, 90, 93, 94, 95
sexually transmitted diseases (STDs), 127
Sketch Engine, 135, 136, 158
social actor representation, 19, 153, 155, 161, 166
social media, 61
statistical measures, 5, 89, 98, 157
stigma, 19, 59, 61, 64, 130, 155
systemic functional linguistics (SFL), 154, 162

transcription, 41, 43, 126, 206
treatment, 88, 90, 149, 150

United Kingdom, 36, 109, 110, 144, 186, 197, 210, 212

vaccination, 46, 119, 120, 124, 177, 212
  anti-vaccination, 46, 47, 118, 170, 173, 179
  human papillomavirus (HPV), 120
  vaccine hesitancy, 46, 120, 124, 170, 176
Van Leeuwen, T., 153, 155, 164, 169
Victorian period, 46, 48, 118, 120

Wmatrix, 106, 145
Word Sketch, 136
WordSmith, 38, 103

For EU product safety concerns, contact us at Calle de José Abascal, 56-1°,
28003 Madrid, Spain or eugpsr@cambridge.org.

www.ingramcontent.com/pod-product-compliance
Ingram Content Group UK Ltd.
Pitfield, Milton Keynes, MK11 3LW, UK
UKHW020142180925
463035UK00020B/597